The Drug Beat

The Drug Beat

by Allen Geller

and Maxwell Boas

McGraw-Hill Book Company
New York St. Louis San Francisco Düsseldorf
Kuala Lumpur Mexico Montreal Panama
Rio de Janeiro Toronto

The Drug Beat

Library of Congress Catalog Card Number 70-78408
Reprinted by arrangement with Cowles Book Company, Inc.
First McGraw-Hill Paperback Edition, 1971
07-023078-1

CONTENTS

Introduction ix
Introduction to the Paperback Edition xv
Glossary xviii

SECTION ONE: MARIJUANA

Chapter 1
The Marijuana Trail: Origins and Early Use. 3
The Smoke from China to Mexico.

Chapter 2
The American Experience: Marijuana in the United States. 15
From the Early Settlers to the Hippies.

Chapter 3
What Is Pot? The Marijuana Plant. 34
Cannabis Sativa and Mary Jane.

Chapter 4
What Pot Does: The Pharmacology of Marijuana. 43
Its Physical and Psychic Effects.

Chapter 5
The Pot Mystique: How Marijuana Is Used. 62
From Copping to the Tea-Pad Party.

Chapter 6
Is Pot Safe? The Medical Picture. 79
The Dangers, the Question of Addiction, the Heroin Problem.

Chapter 7
Pot and the Establishment: The Social Aspects. 95
Crime, Sex, Cigarettes, Autos, and Alcohol.

Chapter 8
Pot and the Authorities: The Legislation. 112
From the Marijuana Menace to LeMar.

Chapter 9
Underground Pot: The Criminal Aspects. 128
From the Mexican Barrios to the American Suburbs.

Chapter 10
Pot and the GI: The Military Scene. 145
The Grass from Panama to Vietnam.

SECTION TWO: LSD

Chapter 11
The First Trip: Blazing the Psychedelic Trail. 155
A Bicycle Ride, Waltzing Mice, and Schizophrenia.

Chapter 12
LSD for Everyone: The Leary-Alpert Complex. 161
Dropouts Turn America on.

Chapter 13
The New Prohibition: Anti-LSD Legislation. 171
The Establishment Versus Flower Power.

Chapter 14
Black-Market Acid: The Threat of the Mafia. 178
Cornering the Underground Acid Market.

Chapter 15
Tuning In: How LSD Works. 187
Preparing to Leave Ground Control.

Chapter 16
Turned On: The Impact of LSD. 197
Altering Senses and Expanding Consciousness.

Chapter 17
Flying High: The Mind Unshackled. 203
The Treasure Trove of the Psyche.

Chapter 18
Acid Therapy: LSD and Mental Health. 214
Neurosis, Psychosis, and Alcoholism.

Chapter 19
A Love Drug: LSD and Sex. 225
From Frigidity to the Marriage Bed.

SECTION THREE: AMPHETAMINES

Chapter 20
Speed Kills: The Abuse of Amphetamines. 233
New Labs—the Family Medicine Cabinet, the Garden, and the Supermarket.

Chapter 21
Methedrine: The Superman Drug. 239
"If Mother Uses It, Can It Be So Bad?"

Chapter 22
The Speed Scene: The Logistics of Meth. 256
Teen-Age Speed Freaks.

Afterword 263

Bibliography 269

Index 271

INTRODUCTION

"The times, they are a-changing," sings Bob Dylan. Another song by this lyrical spokesman for an alienated youth taunts the American Everyman: "Something is happening, but you don't know what it is, do you, Mr. Jones?" Mr. Jones must be given more credit than the song grants him. He knows that what's happening is pot, acid, and speed.

These three drugs share the common characteristic of altering the consciousness to a degree that can range from revelation and euphoria to depression and fear. Sought out by the serious-minded and thrill seeker alike, they are hedged by the most stringent state and federal laws. Yet, paradoxically, their growing consumption is one of America's most wide-open secrets. Unlike such fads as purring with catnip, sniffing airplane glue, and smoking baked banana peels, they are the hard core of the drug revolution sweeping America.

Marijuana, LSD, and amphetamine are vibrations from a transmission center far beyond the wave lengths of conventional communication media. They transport some people while frightening others. And, despite the massive arsenal of legislative curbs, they bridle at control, and whirl into the darkest caverns of the mind. To individuals riding its waves, the mind drug promises instant terror or instant bliss, and sometimes both. No one who has felt or heard these aerial stirrings remains unaffected.

All across America people are tuning in to this new phenomenon. Looking about them, they observe the familiar forms of their environment take on the new shapes and colors that stem directly from the drug experience. Wall posters in psychedelic colors convey their messages in flashes of hallucinogenic insight. Dress is becoming more bizarre, designed to express the individual rather than the dicta of standard tastes. Light machines, stroboscopes, and multiple-projection cinema illuminate the frontiers of the new consciousness. Music originates from as many as a dozen sources at once to overwhelm the ear and pull the listener into a total sense of involvement. Like the tribal joys of adornment for adornment's sake, trinkets, beads, and amulets mock the concepts of decreed taste. "Head" shops and psyche-delicatessens sell incense instead of Air-Wick. Relationships between the sexes are concerned less with the social niceties of the past than with a forthright appreciation of the individual as such. The single dimension in American life is being shattered. As the psychedelic generation matures to play its role in the national life, only one thing is certain: America will never be the same again.

Drugs have helped cleave the generation gap to a width unequalled in any other period of American history. The upheaval of values induced by the use of drugs seems to be closely tied to the new activism revealed in student rebellions, draft resistance, and militant marchers. The belief among the young that they do have the power to pressure, if not change, the world is a phenomenon with close links to the subculture of drugs that is altering old thinking patterns and providing a new perspective on contemporary world issues.

As yet, the majority of this movement burbles underground, surfacing in the form of Flower Children, hippies, and yippies. From San Francisco's Haight-Ashbury to New York's East Village, youngsters are "flipping out" on mysterious wave lengths. Their shrines are mind-bending sanctums—the Electric Circus, the Fillmore, and hundreds of smaller ballrooms and discotheques. The apostles of the supercharged sound of the sixties are telling it like it is—Big Brother and the Holding Company, the Mothers of Invention, Country Joe and the Fish, the Quicksilver Messenger Service.

The "turned-on" generation blows its mind at freak-outs, love-ins, and psychedelic-light shows. To help them arrange the novel insights and experiences, they read ancient Hindu sages, the *I Ching,* the *Tibetan Book of the Dead.* Marijuana and LSD propel them into hitherto unmapped regions of the mind while the mystical lore of the East serves as a guide through this virgin terrain. They have rejected Freudian psychoanalysis, the Western contribution to the exploration of the mind, as inadequate. Their faith reposes in astrologer's charts, gurus, and an uncompromising commitment "to know thyself." A subsequent preoccupation with the East—especially India—has led to the popularity of the meditative retreats known as ashrams, yoga disciplines, and Hare Krishna chants as the more efficacious means of restoring the psyche to an atmosphere of contemplative calm.

The adoption of a life style totally removed from the standard experience has, not unexpectedly, infused the young with an exhilarating sense of self-assurance. They tell frightened elders and perplexed authorities "where it's at." Their key words are "peace" and "love"; violence is countered with Flower Power. A new generation is basing its assumptions on the inner spirit rather than the appearance of things. In less than five years it has pulled the rug from under America's moral foundations.

The most striking illustration of the evolution of a taboo, defined by the most severe punitive legislation, to a practice that has gained a wide measure of respectability is the emergence of marijuana on the national scene. Though still frowned upon by law enforcers, it has progressed from an activity associated mainly with the criminal fringe to the point where it has become a middle-class phenomenon. This shift to the more respectable segments of our population has not escaped the attention of our social satirists. The late Lenny Bruce once remarked that the legalization of pot would not be long in coming for the same law students now smoking it would constitute the vanguard in the fight to make it legal. Already there are signs of changing public attitudes that point to the possibility that current laws that now make smoking pot a punishable offense *may* eventually be removed.

There is no doubt that unhindered access to marijuana is bound to introduce considerable changes, on all levels of society. Without alcohol our environment would be different from what it is today. So the possible emancipation of pot is certain to affect both the substance and quality of life in America. Yet, despite all the prophets of doom, many authorities believe that such a transformation will not necessarily be pejorative.

The sad statistics of alcohol show that its abuse will be with us regardless of the legislation in force. Legalization of marijuana would unquestionably produce a subculture of dropouts and fringe elements; it has already, despite the restrictive laws long in force against it. But at the same time some advocates are convinced that the vast majority of those enjoying the legal right to smoke marijuana will not abuse the privilege. They consider it far more probable that they will exercise restraint and moderation, just as the social drinker limits his indulgence to specific occasions when he feels like having a few "shots." On the other hand, the more hard-headed legislators feel that this assumption would be expecting too much in the light of their experience with drug users.

Unfortunately much of today's opinion concerning marijuana

is still informed by the same reasoning that has led the authorities to classify the drug as a narcotic, which it is not. One would not be unreasonable in stating that, if marijuana hadn't been riddled with legal obstacles to its acquisition, it today might be looked upon with a greater measure of social approval than alcohol. A number of medical studies (among them the Boston University marijuana report) have drawn conclusions supporting the belief that the drug is a harmless product of the milder hallucinogenic variety.

Recently, the drug laws were further complicated by the appearance of a substance that, at the time of its emergence, sounded as innocent as alphabet soup—LSD-25. Whether it is the "least dangerous substance available to man," as Timothy Leary believes, or a threat not only to the user but to unborn generations as well, as Dr. Goddard, former head of the Food and Drug Administration believes, the fact remains that the powerful chemical has become very much a part of the contemporary drug scene. Whereas marijuana could be handled in the light of a certain amount of known factors, the arrival of LSD threw the legislators into a temporary tizzie. Not only was very little known about its mind-changing properties, but its effects were reported to be more far-reaching than any ever claimed for pot.

A complete ban on its use and manufacture soon followed, despite the fact that the exploration of its clinical and therapeutic application was still in its infancy. The LSD cult is more than "kicks" sought by thrill seekers. Its beneficient application in the cure of alcoholism and certain types of schizophrenia is well-known. Beyond that it points to a totally new direction in American life. And LSD continues to flourish in a growing swathe of the American drug culture with results that are already becoming apparent in the psychedelic turn of some of our popular arts and commercial enterprises.

Sociologists view its popularity as a reaction against a stridently materialistic society. The LSD cultist withdraws into his own mind, seeks his own spiritual values, and tries to live accordingly. Communities of LSD users already dot the rural environs of a number of American cities. The cultist simply drops out of the mainstream of American life, centering the world within himself and other community members. The drug's disciples don't look upon their withdrawal as alienation. They claim to be in much closer rapport with their environment than the person whose consciousness has not been expanded by LSD.

Unlike heroin, the use of which nobody sanctions, marijuana, LSD, and the amphetamines have burst upon us with a plethora of defenders and outspoken advocates for their use—from the Beatles to psychologists, philosophers, doctors—all arguing vociferously against the official position. It is this phenomenon—its use and support by a large membership of the respectable middle class—that separates these three drugs so distinctly from the hard narcotics.

Currently, the use of these three drugs is still largely associated with the younger generation, which has stamped its character on the phenomenon just as an earlier generation left its more pathetic mark of the junkie. To today's "heads" the junkie with his aura of defeat and wretched hang-ups is a subject of pity, if not outright scorn. They see him as one gripped in the vise of a habit that has gone out of control, a condition they consider distinctly "uncool." The modern user of hallucinogens thinks his practice has implicit values, not the least of which is a defiance of the "straight" society of limited experience, to whom the expanded consciousness spells anathema and fear.

However, most authorities agree that the power of mind-expanding chemicals is too great to risk its haphazard and indiscriminate use. Reports showing the possibility of chromosome damage, as well as general concurrence on the drug's deleterious effects on the unstable and anxiety-ridden user, are significant aspects of the evidence against it. Over the past years there has been no shortage of newspaper reports about experimenters who "freaked out" as the result of a "bum trip."

In *The Varieties of Psychedelic Experience,* published by Holt, Rinehart, and Winston, Inc., R. E. L. Masters and J. Houston list some of LSD's far-reaching effects: ". . . changes in visual, auditory, tactile, olfactory, gustatory and kinesthetic perception; changes in experiencing time and space; . . . hallucinations; . . . heightened awareness of color; abrupt and frequent mood and affect changes; . . . depersonalization and ego dissolution; dual, multiple, and fragmentized consciousness; . . . enhanced awareness of linguistic nuances; . . . sense of capacity to communicate much better by non-verbal means; . . . concern with philosophical, cosmological, and religious questions; and, in general, apprehension of a world that has slipped the chains of normal, categorical ordering, leading to an intensified interest in self and world and also to a range of responses moving from extremes of anxiety to extremes of pleasure. . . ."

Such a tremendous potential to alter the consciousness made LSD a sure subject of heated debate.

If there is one aspect of the current drug culture that is looked upon with justified foreboding, it is the recent popularity of amphetamines. Commonly known as "speed," the wasting effects of these drugs have raised concern even among users of marijuana and LSD, who recently put up posters in hippie centers with the warning: "Speed Kills."

Many of the runaway youngsters and social dropouts crowding such hippie enclaves as San Francisco's Haight-Ashbury are "meth freaks." Methedrine, besides inducing a state of euphoria and an exhilarating sense of power, also lays waste the body through lack of sleep and loss of appetite. Overindulgence in amphetamines can be lethal, yet measures taken to curb its use have so far been unsuccessful. To the earnest champion of more liberal drug laws, the "speed freak" is an embarrassment who has served to confuse even further the public notion about drugs in general.

The authors of *The Drug Beat* have attempted to create a thorough survey and assessment of the three major drugs now adrift in a growing undertow of American life. Only through such a familiarity with the properties, characteristics, and influence of the drug phenomenon can the reader see, in the light of reason and unprejudiced opinion, a development that already is too strongly entrenched to be merely wished away.

INTRODUCTION TO THE PAPERBACK EDITION

"They ought to lock them kids up." "Dope drives them crazy; they don't know what they're doing." "Those addicts should all be shot."

"Oh, wow, like dope is boss." "Just groovy, you know." "Beautiful, beautiful, beautiful. So beautiful."

Since *The Drug Beat* first appeared the debate has continued to rage—each side condemning or glorifying substances they know little about. What the participants don't realize is that it is too late now. Too late to discuss either in outraged moral tones or unadulterated paeans of praise whether or not we should allow our citizens to ingest drugs with the possibility of coming, finally, to a decision for or against their use. The plain fact is that drug use is firmly established in our society—especially among our younger generation to whom it is as American as apple pie.

Yet while it is cliché to point out that we now live in a drug culture and to repeat such statistics as "close to 100 mood pills were consumed per person last year," there are still those who refuse to see the forest for the trees. They continue to point to the sensational instances of drug abuse that show up in their newspapers and tut-tut what they think the aberration of the few—without acknowledging the unparalleled rise in drug use that has invaded the scrubbed precincts of middle-class America and that has become an increasing worry of medical authorities and social legislators alike.

They think of today's young drug users as having appeared on the scene overnight—some foreign element risen from a dark, ugly cellar and back into which they should immediately be stuffed. But drug use can no longer be associated with only the radical and criminal fringes of society; its implications cover a far wider spectrum. Last year alone there were over 300,000 persons arrested on various drug charges, 60 to 70% of that figure representing pot violations, and nearly all of the arrests were in the 15- to 25-year age group. Needless to say, the arrested are only the tip of the iceberg.

It appears strange only to the very few who shy away from adding any chemical whatsoever to their bloodstream to hear that their neighbor, feeling anxious or angry may pop a tranquilizer, feeling nervous about a social occasion may gulp a martini, or feeling sleepless may swallow a barbiturate at night; or that their son may chew pep pills to cram for an examination. America *is* a drug-oriented society and adults have set the standard by their own behavior.

Today's teenagers entered a world in which mood-changing substances were a fact of existence; sleeping pills, stimulants, tranquilizers, depressants and many other varieties of mind-altering chemical compounds had long been absorbed into the nation's pharmacopoeia, and copping pills, swallowing capsules and downing tablets were a national habit. Our youngsters' indulgence in drugs can hardly be blamed on some sinister outside influence; they witnessed firsthand the tranquilizer–amphetamine–barbiturate boom of the fifties as their own parents took eagerly to psychic delights. They grew up regarding chemicals as tools to be used to manipulate the inner mind. Some youngsters were even recipients of these drugs; until the dangers were clearly delineated, it was not uncommon for parents to dose their children with half a barbiturate tablet so that they would be sure to go to sleep.

Thus reared on a diet of mood-altering drugs along with their Wheaties and sundaes, it was only to be expected that the youngsters would emulate their parents' habits, and it was against the backdrop of drug use in the grown-up world that they, eventually, began sniffing glue and raiding their parents' medicine cabinets to obtain those chemical kicks that their parents seemed to be experiencing. It wasn't really much of a step from that to marijuana as they took their own independent look into other substances. And today pot, acid and speed, though illegal, are widespread enough to be termed "pop drugs."

What is a society to do if millions of its young citizens insist on consuming substances most authorities consider taboo; when they consider these drugs more appropriate to their life styles than the drugs their parents use?

A very serious look must be taken at what's happening. In the last few years the evils that come from the underground, and therefore unregulatable, drug market have been given ample publicity. As well, the shortcomings of restrictive legislation—

resulting in crowded court calendars and tragic waste of young lives, but hardly in curbing the multiplying population of drug consumers—has been made apparent. Yet the role of drugs in this traumatic period of culture clash—their psychic and social consequences—has been little understood. The acrimonious debate goes on but leads nowhere. As *The Drug Beat* tries to point out, it is only in objectively understanding the configuration of forces that we can move toward wiser public policies in the future and hope to influence the ultimate effects upon us.

GLOSSARY

Acapulco Gold: Supposedly the all-time supersmoke of the many different varieties of marijuana tobacco. It compares so favorably to hashish that it sells for as much as $40 an ounce.

Acid: D-lysergic acid diethylamide tartrate, referred to in laboratory shorthand as LSD-25. It is the most powerful of the consciousness-expanding drugs and takes the user on a trip through the psyche. Underground price per trip, $5 to $10. *See* also MIKE.

Acidhead: A frequent user of LSD who takes the drug without any specific motivation except for thrills. *See* also HEAD.

Aimies: The amphetamine group of stimulants including benzedrine, dexedrine, and methedrine. The effects of *aimies* are said to resemble those of a very low dose of cocaine. They generate a pleasurable, expansive, and benevolent mood as well as feelings of superiority, elation, and excitement. They also offer relief from fatigue, which is the reason for their frequent use among truckdrivers. They are also used in reducing programs and as antidepressants. *See* also BENNY, CRYSTAL, DEXIES, SPEED, and UPPIES.

Amphetamines: *See* AIMIES.

Bag: (1) The envelope in which a drug is packaged, usually the size of a conventional tea bag. (2) The thing you care about most, that which expresses one's personality and attitude. "Music is my bag." *See* also DO YOUR THING.

Bail of Hay: A bulky amount of marijuana, so-called because it is difficult to flush down the toilet—the usual way to get rid of it in case of emergency.

Banana: The fruit purportedly acts as a mild hallucinogenic when baked and crumbled and rolled into a cigarette.

Bar: A quantity of marijuana in block shape, usually smuggled into the country. Gum arabic or honey is often used as a binding agent.

Beat: Down low, used to describe a dropout who has not turned on and tuned in. *See* also TURN ON, TURN IN, DROP OUT.

Bee: A measure of marijuana approximately the size of a penny match box.

Benny: Benzedrine, a stimulant in the amphetamine group generally taken in tablet or capsule form but sometimes injected. It is also used in nasal inhalers for colds. The effects are euphoric but usage dropped considerably with the introduction of dexedrine, a more powerful stimulant. *See* also AIMIES, CRYSTAL, DEXIES.

Bhang: An Indian variety of cannabis composed of the flowering tops, leaves, and resin of both male and female plants. It is slightly stronger than the American marijuana.

Blast: To smoke marijuana.

Blow: To smoke a marijuana cigarette.

Bomb: An unusually large or thick marijuana cigarette.

Bombed out: High on marijuana or any other drug.

Bombitas: Slang for methedrine. *See also* SPEED.

Boo: Marijuana.

Boo-Hoo: High priest of the neo-American Church, which uses marijuana and psychedelic drugs as sacraments.

Boss: An adjective meaning "great" or "good." "Boss pot" means good marijuana.

Bread: Money. *See* also CHANGE, SMASH.

Brick: A kilogram (2.2 pounds) of marijuana.

Bummer: A bad deal or a bad *trip* on LSD.

Burned: To get cheated in a drug deal.

Bust: Arrest for violation of drug laws.

Cancelled Stick: (a) A regular tobacco cigarette, also known as a *square.* The *cancelled stick* may be emptied of its contents and filled with marijuana. (2) A bad marijuana cigarette.

Cannabis sativa. Indian hemp plant that yields marijuana, hashish, and *ganja.*

Cannibinol: Chemically isolated resin of *Cannabis sativa.*

Change: Money. *See* also BREAD, SMASH.

Charas: Another cannabis extract found primarily in India. It is about eight times as powerful as ordinary marijuana.

Chillum: Cylindrical pipe through which marijuana is smoked by sucking at its narrow bottom. Its use has spread from India to the more knowledgeable smokers in the United States.

Chucks: The hunger that often follows the smoking of marijuana. The intense craving for food is also sometimes referred to as a *peppermint candy jag.*

Clean: Being free of any evidence of carrying marijuana or other drugs. Also the removal of all extraneous matter, such as stems, stalks, seeds, from marijuana prior to smoking it.

Cocktail: The short butt of a marijuana cigarette inserted into a regular cigarette when it becomes too small to be held comfortably for smoking.

Connection: The contact man who supplies marijuana or other drugs.

Cook: To boil a solution of a drug, especially if the drug is suspected of being *turd* (impure). This is usually done with a spoon and a match.

Cop: To buy or obtain drugs. To "cop a bag" is to get hold of a bag of marijuana or other drugs.

Co-pilot: The person with whom one takes the *trip.*

Crash: The pleasurable sleep following the smoking of marijuana.

Crutch: A simple device used to hold a short marijuana cigarette. It can be anything from a hair clip to tweezers.

Crystal: Methedrine, the superpowerful pep drug in the amphetamine group favored by hippies. Medically employed as an antidepressant, it is similarly used by the hippies, who also take it with marijuana to insure a better *high.* Recently some *acid* has been cut with *crystal* to stimulate the flash lacking in low-quality *acid. See* also FLASH.

Dealer: Seller of marijuana and drugs.

Destroyed: Worn out, exhausted, from the use of drugs.

Dexie: Dexedrine, a stimulant in the amphetamine group. Effects are similar to benzedrine but more powerful and without certain side effects. Like benzedrine, which it once replaced, it is now being supplanted by methedrine, the new superamphetamine. They are cheap: A couple cost but a penny at the drugstore and anywhere from a nickel to a quarter per tablet on the street. *See* also BENNY, CRYSTAL.

Dippie: A onetime hippie who dropped out of the movement and into *straight* society.

Djamba: Also known as *dagga,* it is a somewhat stronger African form of cannabis.

Down: To be in a low emotional state. The effects of a drug produce a *high.* To *come down* describes the feeling of depression after the effects of the drugs have worn off. To *put down* generally refers to being hostile to another.

Downies: Drugs that depress as opposed to drugs that stimulate, especially barbiturates and narcotics. Since *downies* inhibit mental activity, *hippies* use them when trying to *come down.* The narcotics are not too popular among the *hippies,* and the barbiturates (e.g. phenobarbital) have a dangerous soporific effect. *See* UPPIES, SMACK.

Do Your Thing: To lead a private, personalized way of life that *grooves* you and *turns you on.* Hippie philosophy holds that you don't try to force your *thing* on anyone else. On this basis a few hippie zealots were persuaded to abandon their idea of polluting San Francisco's water system with enough LSD to *turn on* the rest of the city.

Drop out: The last step in the *turn-on, tune-in, drop-out* cycle. To detach oneself from what hippies consider the regimented, stultifying, dog-eat-dog games of the *straight* world. What one drops *into* is *doing your thing. See* also TURN ON, TUNE IN.

Dynamite: Superior marijuana or any potent mind-affecting drug.

Explorers' Club: Group of *acidheads.*

Flash: The first sensation immediately after taking the drug. Low-grade *acid* is sometimes adulterated with methedrine to heighten the initial *flash.*

Flip out: To lose one's control and self-possession while under the influence of a drug. It also describes an overwhelming reaction to something particularly striking.

Floating: A feeling of intoxication through smoking marijuana.

Flower Power: The moral force exerted by hippies in dealing with unfriendly or hostile elements. A passive approach seeking a reconciliation of differences through love.

Fly: The sensation felt when using the uppies and psychedelics; also used as an adjective meaning "good." *See* HEAVY.

Flying: To be extremely *high* on pot or other drugs.

Freak: (1) A heavy user of drugs. (2) A term applying to both *hip* and *unhip* persons that can be used in a flattering as well as a pejorative sense.

Freak out: To become so completely engrossed in *doing your thing* that contact with the external world is lost. If on drugs, it means so *high* that one is in agony or on the verge of losing control of oneself.

Freaky: Something that is scarifying, weird, strange.

Fuzz: The police. Other terms include the "Feds" for federal agents; "locals" for local authorities. The "people" is a New Orleans expression referring specifically to narcotics agents.

Fuzz Fear: A paranoia sometimes produced by smoking marijuana in which the smoker believes that the authorities are about to arrest him. In this state everyone appears to be some kind of policeman in disguise aware of the smoker's condition.

Gage (Gauge): Marijuana.

Ganja: A specific Indian cannabis product somewhat stronger than regular marijuana.

Geeze: To inject a drug intravenously. *See* MAINLINE.

Golden Leaf: Good-quality marijuana.

Goof (on): To *play with someone's head,* that is, *to put him on* in an attempt to break down his reserve or find out what kind of person he is.

Gopher: Someone who will *go for* a pickup when the buyer is from another area and doesn't know the *pusher.*

Grass: The currently popular term for marijuana that replaces pot, which supplanted "weed," "tea," "bobo bush," "gage," "ginga," "griffa," "hay," "hemp," "Mary Jane," "loco weed," etc. *Cannabis indica* is the pharmaceutical term referring specifically to the resin from the leaves and other tissues of the Indian hemp plant that produce the effect of the drug.

Great Mantra: Slow, hynotic Buddhist chant either sung or listened to by hippies when *flying* on acid. It is also common as part of the setting for a psychedelic session.

Groovy: Smooth, without transition and discordancy. Something is *groovy* when it leads to following one's thoughts, actions, or sensations.

Guru: A Hindu spiritual guide, but among drug users someone who has taken many *trips* and is therefore an excellent guide to the less experienced.

Hash: Hashish, the nearly pure resin of the hemp plant and flowers, five to ten times more potent than regular marijuana tobacco. Hash is smoked in tiny-bowled pipes with long bamboo stems similar in shape to the American Indian peace pipe.

Hashbury: Short for Haight-Ashbury, the locale of two intersecting San Francisco streets and the focal point of the hippie movement on the West Coast. The largest hippie "ghetto" in the world.

Hay: Marijuana.

Head: Generic term for the frequent user of marijuana. Differentiations are made in the kinds of *heads,* such as *potheads, speedheads* (amphetamine users) and *acidheads* (LSD users).

Heavy: Narcotic drugs—morphine, cocaine, and heroin—as opposed to the psychedelic drugs—LSD, psilocybin, mescaline, peyote, marijuana.

High: The euphoric state induced by any mind-altering substances, from marijuana to alcohol.

Hip: To be *turned on* and *tuned in;* to know the score. To be *hip* doesn't necessarily mean that one has to drop out of *straight* society.

Hippie: A spiritual dropout from society who refuses to adopt the Establishment values.

Hit: The drug's effect on the consciousness, sometimes called a "buzz." To get a *hit* is to experience a concrete pleasurable sensation as a result of using the drug. *See* FLASH.

Holding: Being in possession of any drug.

Hookah: Water pipe of the Eastern variety used to smoke marijuana. It is also known as a "hubble-bubble."

Jag: State of extreme stimulation produced by marijuana or other drugs. A "laughing jag" is one of such effects.

Joint: Marijuana cigarette, also referred to as a "stick," "reefer," "weed," "muggles," "rocket," and "twist." Usually hand-rolled, it is about half as thick as an ordinary cigarette. King-size (*see* BOMB) is as big or bigger than an ordinary cigarette. The *joint* generally sells for 25¢ to 50¢ depending on the size of the cigarette and quality of tobacco. Marijuana bags or match boxes run from $5 to $10.

Karma: Buddhist principle of fate or destiny. Many of the serious-minded drug users prefer to control their own *Karma* rather than have it dictated by what they consider the distorted values of the *straight* world.

Key: A kilogram of marijuana.

Kief: Middle Eastern variety of cannabis.

Lid: An ounce of marijuana.

Light Show: A simultaneous projection of light-and-film effects superimposed on one another for the purpose of creating a mind-bending whole. Frequently used as a backdrop for acid-rock groups, it may also be used at home to create the setting of an LSD trip.

Light up: To smoke marijuana.

Lippie: A hippie preoccupied with putting down *straight* society. Many of today's black humorists are referred to by this term.

Mainline: To inject a drug intravenously. *See* GEEZE.

Man: The police or any law enforcer. Negroes use this term to refer to the white man; to someone on the job it means the boss.

Mary Jane: Marijuana.

Meth: Methedrine, one of the most powerful amphetamines. *See* SPEED.

Mike: A microgram or gamma, constituting one millionth of a gram; 250 *mikes* of LSD (1/100,000 of an ounce), the usual dose, is a minute amount of the drug but nevertheless enough to induce the *acid trip.*

Mishwacan: A potent variety of marijuana from Mexico's Morelia district prized by West Coast smokers.

Nark: Narcotics agent.

Nickel Bag: Five dollars' worth of marijuana.

Nutmeg: Long known as a euphoriant among sailors and prisoners who used it for lack of anything more stimulating, the spice was recently found to contain a small amount of hallucinogenic material. It produces acute nausea, vomiting, vertigo, general delirium, and perhaps a few flashes of psychedelic insight; considered highly dangerous.

Panama Red. Also known as "P.R.," it is a reddish form of cannabis found in Panama; extremely popular among connoisseurs. It is expensive: $30 an ounce.

Peace: The operative word in the hippie jargon, it is sometimes used as a greeting, but most commonly stands for the frame of mind aspired to by those who *turn on.*

Peppermint Candy Jag: The hunger for sweets caused by smoking marijuana, especially among younger smokers. *See* CHUCKS.

Periwinkle. The dried and shredded leaves of a blue-blossomed plant common throughout the United States, which when smoked produces a mild type of psychedelic *high.*

Pin: A thin marijuana cigarette.

Plastics: The weekend or phony hippies who flock to hippie communities for short periods but are neither serious smokers nor in sympathy with hippie philosophy.

Pop: To inject a drug. *See* SKIN POP.

Pot: The current term for marijuana, supplanting the "tea" and "weed" of the forties and fifties.

Pusher: The contact who sells *pot* or drugs.

Reefer: A marijuana cigarette.

Riff: (1) Your *thing* or bag. (2) To *groove,* to be in tune and enjoying one's friends or environment.

Roach: The butt of a marijuana cigarette, usually smoked in such contraptions as *cocktails, steamboats,* and *zooies.*

Rush: The first euphoric effects after taking a drug. *See* also FLASH.

Salt and Pepper: Adulterated marijuana. A typical adulterate is catnip, which looks and smells like *grass.*

Scag: (1) An *unhip* person, a "jerk." (2) Pejorative name used by potheads for heroin addicts. (3) Heroin.

Score: To succeed in obtaining or buying pot or drugs.

Seed: The butt of a marijuana cigarette or the seed of the cannabis plant usually found among the tobacco; too many seeds indicate an inferior quality of marijuana.

Set: The frame of a person's mind prior to taking LSD or smoking pot.

Setting: The total environment conductive to the LSD experience. Lights, music, and art objects are considered necessary props to a pleasant and meaningful trip.

Shades: Dark glasses worn to hide the effects of LSD and marijuana on the eyes (pupillary dilation, pinkish whites, and baggy lids).

Sitar: Indian instrument in the shape of a lute with long neck; popular for background music during psychedelic sessions.

Skin: Cigarette paper used for rolling marijuana.

Skin Pop: Injection of a drug not directly into a vein to slow down the drug's effects and produce a more pleasurable *high.*

Smack: Heroin, also known as "scag," "H," "horse," and "Henry." Although not very popular among serious smokers, it is sometimes used as a means to *come down* from *flying too high* on *crystal.*

Smash: Money. *See* BREAD, CHANGE.

Snoops: Detectives; undercover narcotics agents.

Space: To live without encumbrance of any sort. To live freely by one's wits or by the charity of others.

Speed: The amphetamines, benzedrine, dexedrine, but particularly methedrine (*crystal*). Use of these drugs gives an illusion of power and action and frequently brings on catatonic effects—glazed eyes, jerky movements, rapid heartbeat, and bizarre mental effects.

Speed Freak: One who overindulges in the use of amphetamines, especially methedrine.

Spike: The hypodermic needle used to inject drugs.

Splash: Amphetamines. *See* SPEED.

Spring: To treat a person to a *toke* on a marijuana cigarette.

Square: A regular tobacco cigarette.

Stash: (1) A hidden supply of marijuana. (2) Its hiding place.

Steamboat: A *roach*-holding device made from an empty toilet roll. The *roach* is put into a small hole in the cylinder, thus resembling the smoke stack on a steamboat. One end is covered with the palm of one hand and the open end of the cylinder is used for inhaling.

Stick: A marijuana cigarette.

Stoned: The sensation of being *high* on drugs.

STP: A newly developed hallucinogenic drug supposedly fifty times as powerful as LSD.

Straight: A person who doesn't smoke pot; a "square."

Strung out: Exhausted, usually through use of drugs, especially methedrine.

Sugar Cube: A dose of LSD in sugar-cube form.

Synhexyl: A synthetic preparation of the active principle of the marijuana drug.

Tab: An LSD pill. One *tab* may contain more than one *trip.*

Tabla: Indian drum, sometimes used as part of the setting of the LSD trip.

Taste: A small amount of drugs usually just enough for one person's use.

Tea: Marijuana.

Tetrahydrocannabinol: Cannabis substance that has been synthesized into the form of a marijuana pill.

Thumb: A thick marijuana cigarette.

Toke: A pull at a marijuana cigarette. To *toke up* is to light up a *joint.*

Travel Agent: The LSD connection; supplier of LSD.

Trip: The actual psychedelic experience, so-called because under the influence of LSD one "travels" to unknown and unexpected places.

Tune-in: The frame of mind conducive to illuminating society at large; the refusal to accept society on its own terms.

Turd: A drug of low potency or high adulteration.

Turn on: One may *turn* on in a variety of ways—through hallucinogens, *grass,* religious chants, sex, or any other consciousness-expanding experience. LSD is most favored. According to its advocates, LSD deconditions the mind and leads its users to a greater confidence in individual experience and intuitive feelings. *See* also DROP OUT, TUNE IN.

Twisted: The state of mind induced by drugs, resulting in a complete loss of the ego sense and accepted norms of behavior.

Up Front: Money given on trust to a person for marijuana before the actual purchase takes place.

Uppies: Any stimulant, such as the amphetamines, that increases mental activity. *See* also DOWNIES, AIMIES.

Vibrations: The invisible extensions of one's surroundings or activity. *Vibrations* emanating from an experience, such as listening to music or seeing a film, are considered by the turned-on generation a basis for judgment. Feeling, rather than intellectual appreciation, is emphasized.

Wasted: Worn out, usually as a result of taking drugs.

Weight: (1) A large amount of any drug. (2) Any amount of a certain drug, as in "Are you carrying any *weight*?"

Works: The needle, eye dropper, spoon, or any other device needed for intravenous injection of a drug, usually heroin or methedrine.

Yippie: Successor to the hippie. The yippie is more action-minded—politically and otherwise.

Zooie: A *roach*-smoking device made by rolling an empty matchbook cover into a cylinder, thus forming a miniature cigarette holder.

SECTION ONE:

MARIJUANA

CHAPTER ONE

THE MARIJUANA TRAIL: ORIGINS AND EARLY USE

The Smoke from China to Mexico

Marijuana is only one of the many terms used for the various intoxicating preparations produced from the Indian hemp plant. Cannabis, *bhang, kif, hashish,* pot, charge, tea, *ganja,* and grass are some of the other names associated with the drug. The Bureau of Narcotics alone keeps a list of more than three hundred different terms.

Indian hemp has been known to man for more than five thousand years. Although originally indigenous to Central Asia, the plant is now found in practically every section of the world, where it either grows wild or is cultivated legally and otherwise. *Cannabis sativa*—the technical term for the plant—has been known in India and the Middle East since time immemorial. It was a favorite of yogis and other religious contemplatives who used it to still the distractions of their environment.

How far back the plant itself goes has not been determined, but it was first mentioned in a monograph written in 2737 B.C. by the Chinese Emperor Shen Neng. The intoxicating qualities of the resin of the plant had probably been discovered by accident as people inhaled the smoke from burning hemp. Since Shen Neng's is the earliest account of the drug and its strange effects, one can only guess at how long the Chinese cultivated it before stumbling on its use as an intoxicant. Norman Taylor, in his book, *Narcotics: Nature's Dangerous Gifts,* mentions that records from the court of Shen Neng show that the plant was raised for its fibers, which the Chinese used to manufacture a wide range of clothing.

Besides using *cannabis* as a commercial staple and intoxicant, the Chinese applied it to the practice of medicine soon after they discovered its pharmaceutical qualities. Emperor Shen Neng gave authoritative proof that the Chinese found it to be an effective anesthetic in surgery. He looked into its possible applications, just as in our age researchers carried out experiments with the drug's medicinal powers until its ban in this country. Throughout history cannabis has had a wide use in indigenous medicine, especially in India, and to some extent in modern medicine. Today, however, its unsavory reputation has largely stymied further research.

Documentation of the wide-spread use of cannabis for medical, religious, and intoxicant purposes begins to appear in about the tenth century B.C. when the peoples of Asia and Africa began to use the drug in a rather indiscriminate manner. The Greek historian Herodotus (about 484-425 B.C.), writes of how the Scythians—the early inhabitants of what is now a mountainous region of Siberia in Soviet Russia—got intoxicated on cannabis by throwing the hemp seeds onto a bed of ashes and hot stones and inhaling the smoke.

In India the cannabis plant was cultivated specifically for the drug obtained from the resin. It is mentioned repeatedly in ancient Indian literature. The fourth book of the Vedas in Hindu literature refers to the drug as a "Bringer of Happiness," while other Indian descriptions of cannabis preparations were extant as early as 2000 B.C.

Cannabis was used in Indian religious rituals to "clear the head and stimulate the brain to think" during meditation. According to two medical authorities who have been studying drug usage in India for years, R. N. and G. S. Chopra, "the deliberate abuse of *bhang* [cannabis] is met with almost entirely among certain classes of religious mendicants." This shows clearly that from its first mention in Hindu religious literature the use of cannabis eventually spread to all classes of Indian society. Such indulgence is today frowned upon by the Indian upper and middle classes despite the fact that the practice was held in great esteem in ancient times.

The Chopra brothers report that its use has gradually declined —especially over the past thirty years—and at "the present time is almost entirely confined to the lower strata of society." They put current usage at only twenty-five percent of what was consumed in the country at the turn of the century—a decline they attribute largely to a higher excise duty on the cannabis crop that has reduced the areas under cultivation. This percentage, however, makes up a considerable portion of world-wide usage, estimated at 200 million by a United Nations-sponsored survey in 1950. With its users largely concentrated in Africa and Asia, the United Nations figure makes cannabis, next to alcohol, the world's second most popular intoxicant.

Although to a lesser extent than previously, the use of cannabis continues to flourish in India. The Indian lower classes, specifically the workingman, today uses cannabis the way beer is consumed in the United States. It is common practice among construction laborers to have a few pulls at a *ganja* (cannabis) pipe or sip a glass of *bhang* (cannabis tea) toward evening. This produces a sense of well-being, relieves fatigue, stimulates the appetite, and induces a feeling of mild stimulation, enabling the worker to bear more cheerfully the strain and monotony of his daily routines.

The drug's popularity as an intoxicant spread from India to the Middle East and in a few centuries had thoroughly impregnated Islamic culture. Moslems readily accepted it as a substitute for alcohol, which is outlawed by their religion. Even so, use of the drug as an intoxicant remained limited among the followers of Mohammed, although Arab doctors employed preparations of cannabis in the cure of a variety of ailments. It was not until the Crusades that the Moslems put the pleasure-giving properties of the plant to wider use. The adverse publicity that has plagued cannabis ever since stems from this period in history.

Marco Polo was the first to convey the bizarre workings of cannabis to the Western world. One of the more striking tales the Venetian traveler brought back from his journeys concerned a doughty Moslem warrior by the name of Hasan-I-Sabbah. Known as the "Old Man of the Mountain," he commanded a stronghold on the craggy peak of Alamut where he kept an army of young warriors who were not unfamiliar with the delights of cannabis.

Hasan, according to the legend, customarily supplied his followers with hashish. For the glimpse of paradise afforded by the drug, his fanatical henchmen would endure any hardship. Riding across the desert to Basra or Baghdad, their one thought was of the glorious reward awaiting them upon completion of their murderous tasks. The words "assassin" and "hashish," for the drug prepared from cannabis, are both supposedly derived from "Hasan," whose men were known in their day as *Thugs* and *Hashishans*. Marco Polo presented this bloody corner of the Moslem world with all the color and pageantry the Europeans of his day associated with the East:

> In the territory of the Assassins there are delicious walled gardens in which one can find everything that can satisfy the needs of the body and the caprices of the most exacting sensuality. Great banks of gorgeous flowers and bushes covered with fruit stand amongst crystal rivers of living water. . . . Trellises of roses and fragrant vines cover with their foliage pavilions of jade or porcelain furnished with Persian carpets and Grecian embroideries.
>
> Delicious drinks in vessels of gold or crystal are served by young boys or girls, whose dark unfathomable eyes cause them to resemble the Houris, divinities of that Paradise which the Prophet promised to believers. The sound of harps mingles with the cooing of doves, the murmur of soft voices blends with the sighing of the reeds. All is joy, pleasure, voluptuousness and enchantment.
>
> The Grand Master of the Assassins, whenever he discovers a young man resolute enough to belong to his murderous legions, hashish. Having been secretly transported to the pleasure gardens invites the youth to his table and intoxicates him with the plant "hashish." Having been secretly transported to the pleasure gardens the young man imagines that he has entered the Paradise of Mahomet. The girls, lovely as Houris, contribute to the illusion. After he has enjoyed to satiety all the joys promised by the Prophet to his elect, he falls again into a state of lethargy and is transported back to the presence of the Grand Master. Here he is informed that he can enjoy perpetually the delights he has just tasted if he will take part in the war of the Infidel as commanded by the Prophet.

Although recent scholarship has exploded the tale Marco Polo brought back from the East as a myth, and the deviltries supposedly committed by Hasan-I-Sabbah have been proven to be at best an imaginative embellishment of the actual events, translations of the *Arabian Nights,* or *The Thousand and One Nights,* make repeated mention of *benji* (hashish). This intoxicant accompanied the Arabs into Spain in the tenth century. The Arabs, however, confined its use mainly to themselves and it never did become a European habit. When the invading Arabs left Spain, hashish returned along with them to Africa, leaving Europeans with the myth of a magical Eastern drug.

With Napoleon's venture into Egypt at the beginning of the nineteenth century, European interest in the plant was rekindled as returning French soldiers and scientists brought back samples of cannabis. Some medical research into the nature of the drug took place, but the most extensive illumination at the time was produced by the intellectuals and writers who began experimenting with hashish. Popular interest was inflamed by the highly romanticized reports of its marvelous properties that stylishly circulated among the boulevardiers of mid-nineteenth-century Paris.

The intrigue of the East stimulated French thought further as the country proceeded with its colonization of Africa. Exposure to the Arab culture led, among other things, to a study of the religious and sociological aspects of hashish. Unable to abandon their intellectual prejudices, these early investigators concluded that physical and mental deterioration inevitably followed indulgence in the drug. A small minority of artists and less orthodox men of science, however, continued to extol its benefits.

The French Romantic writers were among the drug's most ardent supporters. They wrote expansively about their experiences with the Eastern import and soon formed a group given to experimenting with hashish, called the *Club des Hachischins*. Founded in the mid-nineteenth century by the poets Charles Baudelaire and Théophile Gautier, the club met at the Hotel Pimodan in Paris' Latin Quarter. At that time legal restrictions had not yet been introduced and the club members found themselves free to smoke as much as they liked.

Shortly afterward, however, the French colonialists began to clamp down on the hashish dens in Egypt, pushing the smokers there into underground haunts. But despite this official opprobrium, one member of the *Club des Hachischins*—Dr. Moreau de Tours—returned from Algeria with a good supply of a local delicacy known as *dawamesk,* a mash made up of hemp-plant tops, sugar, orange juice, cinnamon, cloves, cardamon, nutmeg, musk, pistachios, and pine kernels. It sometimes contained a "pinch" of cantharides (a potent poison), which was added to increase the supposed aphrodisiac effect of the mixture. It was this *dawamesk* that created Baudelaire's "artificial paradise," although it is more than likely that his indulgence far exceeded that of smokers today.

Medical authorities agree that an analysis of the literature produced by the club members refers in most cases to experiences with toxic drugs. A review of their drug experiences indicates that the large amounts of hashish they ingested could have caused psychotic episodes and even death. It is certain that sustained use of the dosages they took would result in physical and mental deterioration.

Although the French writers seemed to relish the drug experience, the public who read their literature was of a different mind. The experiences were frightening and repugnant to the bourgeois mentality of the time. As a result the smoking of hashish remained the sub rosa province of a few European artists until the recent trans-Atlantic phenomenon of the American drug culture.

To the members of the *Club*, hashish was the key to the "artificial Paradise." They sang its praises in a body of literature that was for a long period the only work describing the effects of the drug on a number of mental and emotional levels. They were aware that since ancient times artists had used it as a perch from which to launch the imagination. It performed a similar function for the *Hachischins,* except that their interest stemmed more from curiosity about the actual effects than a desire to create literature as such, although incidentally they did that, too.

Baudelaire's book on his experiences with drugs, *The Artificial Paradise,* is one of the finest works on the subject—one he was more than qualified to write. Just one look at the famous photograph on the flyleaf of his works, showing the poet's gaunt face with the sunken eyes and cheeks, the deep lines and bitter lips, lends ready credence to the general belief that he died as a syphilitic wreck, addicted to both opium and alcohol. Nevertheless, the descriptions he gives of his hashish experiences are the least embellished and the most objective of all the writings on the subject by the members of the club.

Baudelaire characterized the hallucinations he underwent as transformations of the real world rather than the creation of an unreal internal world. Similar to the effects ascribed to LSD, his hallucinations seemed to be progressive and almost voluntary, expanding only through the action of the imagination. In *The Artificial Paradise* he first analyzes the "taste for the infinite"—the force in man that drives him beyond the everyday, the force that drives him to indulge in hashish:

Those who are able . . . note in the observatory of their thoughts strange seasons, luxurious afternoons, delicious minutes. There are days when a man awakens with a young and vigorous genius. Hardly have his eyelids cast off the sleep which sealed them before the outer world presents itself to him in strong relief, with a clearness of contour and wealth of admirable color. The man gratified with this sense of exquisite loveliness, unfortunately so rare and so transitory, feels himself more than ever the artist, more than ever noble, more than ever just, if one can express so much in so few words. But the most singular thing about this exceptional state of the spirit and of the senses, which without exaggeration can be termed paradisiacal as compared with the hopeless darkness of ordinary daily existence, is that it has not been created by any visible or easily definable cause.

This acuity of thought, this vigor of sense and spirit, has at all times appeared to man as the highest good. For this reason, purely for his immediate enjoyment, without troubling himself about the limitations imposed by his constitution, he has searched in the world of physical and of pharmaceutical science, among the grossest decoctions and the most subtle perfumes, in all climates and at all times, for the means of leaving, if only for a few moments, his habitation of mud and of transporting himself to Paradise in a single swoop.

Alas! Man's vices, horrible as they are supposed to be, contain the positive proof of his taste for the Infinite. *Man will never believe that he has entirely given himself over to evil.* He forgets, in his infatuation, that he is playing with someone stronger and keener than himself, and that the spirit of Evil, even if one gives it no more than a single hair, will eventually carry away the head. Therefore this visible lord of visible nature (I speak of man) desired to create Paradise with the help of pharmacy, exactly like a maniac who would replace his solid furniture and real gardens with decorations printed on canvas and mounted on easels. I believe that in this depraved sense of the Infinite lies the reason for all guilty excesses, from the solitary and concentrated intoxication of the man of letters who, obliged to turn to opium for relief of some physical suffering, little by little makes it . . . the sum of his spiritual life, to the drunkard who, his brain afire with glory, hideously wallows in the filth of a Paris street.

In the next chapter of *The Artificial Paradise,* entitled "The Theater of the Seraphim," Baudelaire examines the character of the cannabis experience, declaring that it is not one of unnatural visions but rather an exaggeration of the individual's imagination and thoughts. He states that the drug does not destroy the smoker's personality but instead mirrors and enlarges its contours before the mind's eye:

> Ignorant people suppose that the intoxication of hashish represents a prodigious land, a vast theatre of jugglery, in which all is miraculous and unexpected. That is a prejudice, a complete mistake . . . In the intoxication of hashish there is nothing of the kind. Our dreams are natural, our intoxication will always keep the peculiar tonality of the individual. Men who are eager to experience unusual pleasures should know that in hashish they find nothing miraculous, absolutely nothing but what is extremely natural. The brain and the organism on which hashish operates give only their ordinary individual phenomena, increased it is true as to number and energy but always faithful to their origin. Man cannot escape the fatality of his physical and moral temperament. Hashish will be for man's familiar thoughts and impressions a mirror that exaggerates but always a mirror. . . .

In the next section of his book, the poet proceeds to outline a method for taking the drug amazingly similar to Dr. Timothy Leary's prescribed conditions of "set" and "setting." Baudelaire informs the reader of the appropriate frame of mind and environment for the drug experience:

> I presume that you have chosen the right moment for this expedition. Every perfect debauch requires perfect leisure. Besides, hashish not only magnifies the individual but also the circumstance and environment. You must have no duties to accomplish that require punctuality or exactitude, no pangs of love, no domestic preoccupations, griefs, anxieties. The memories of duty will sound a death knell through your intoxication and poison your pleasure. Anxiety will change to anguish, grief to torture. But if the conditions are right and the weather is good, if you are in a favorable environment as in the midst of a picturesque landscape or in a room artistically decorated, if, moreover you can hope to hear some music, then all's for the best.

Baudelaire now outlines four stages of the cannabis experience. The notes emphasize that the members of the *Club des Hachischins* must have taken very large doses indeed for this mildest of hallucinogens to have had these classic effects that so closely resemble that of the much more potent hallucinogen—LSD.

The French poet first describes the anticipation of waiting for the effects to occur and then—the first stage—the breakdown of logical thought patterns, leading to an appreciation of the incongruity of appearances:

> Most novices, during the first step of their initiation, complain of the slow effects of hashish. Then, like the signs of an approaching storm, comes a certain hilarity, irresistible, ludicrous. The simple words, the most trivial ideas take on new and strange shapes, incongruous resemblances and associations impossible to foresee, interminable puns, comical absurdities, rush continually through your brain. From time to time you laugh at yourself, at your foolishness and your folly, and your friends, if you have any, laugh just as boisterously at their condition and your own, but, as they are without malice, you bear no rancor.

Next, Baudelaire gives a very accurate account of the physical effects of the drug—from the coldness felt in the extremities to the dilation of the pupils. These physical symptoms are the second stage. He then goes on to describe the third stage—the stage of expanded consciousness. Although, as mentioned previously, he most probably attained the described effects with inordinately large doses of hashish, it is unlikely that similar results can be achieved with marijuana, the weakest preparation of cannabis. These are effects commonly attained with the more powerful hallucinogens—peyote, mescaline, psilocybin, and LSD:

> It is at this period of the intoxication that a new sensitiveness, a superior acuteness manifests itself in all the senses. Smell, sight, hearing, touch, participate equally in this improvement. The eyes have a vision of Eternity. The ear hears almost inaudible sounds in the midst of a vast tumult. It is then that the hallucinations begin. Exterior objects slowly and successively assume singular appearances; they become deformed and transformed. Then the equivocations commence, the errors and the transposition of ideas. Sounds take on colors and colors contain music. This, one might say, is quite natural, and any poetical mind in a sane and normal

state easily imagines such analogies. But I have already warned the reader that there is nothing supernatural in the intoxication by hashish. These analogies merely assume an unusual vivacity; they penetrate, they invade, they overpower the mind because of their despotic nature.

The altering of the five senses, the crossover of perceptions, the increased sensitivity, the diminished sense of ego, the duality of self, all described by Baudelaire, are amazingly similar to the effects of a good dose of LSD. Although they must have been overpowering effects to control, the French poet retains a scientific view of the occurrences throughout—an amazing detachment, considering the lack of psychological knowledge at the time. He is careful to distinguish between the altered reality of the hashish hallucinations and true hallucinations—a point only recently made by modern-day psychologists in dealing with the complete range of hallucinogens from marijuana to LSD.

Baudelaire, in the chapter of his book entitled "The Man-God," describes the fourth and last stage of the hashish experience—a stage very difficult to achieve even with LSD. It is the state variously called a religious experience, *satori,* a feeling of oneness with God and the universe—the point at which the individual is overcome with joy and good will.

Now my imaginary man, the spirit of my choice, has reached that peculiar state of joy and serenity in which he finds himself *compelled* to admire himself. All contradictions disappear, all philosophical problems become clear or at least seem to. All is food for pleasure. A voice speaks inside him and says to him, "You now have the right to consider yourself superior to all men; no one knows or could understand all that you think and all that you feel; they would even be incapable of appreciating the good will with which they inspired you. You are a king unrecognized by the crowd and who lives alone in his belief; but who cares? Do you not possess a sovereign contempt that strengthens the soul?"

. . . None now should be astonished by the final, the supreme thought born in the dreamer's mind—"I have become God!" That ardent, savage cry bursts from his lips with so intense an energy, with so tremendous a power of projection, that, if the will and belief of an intoxicated man had effective virtue, the cry would topple the very angels scattered about along the roads of heaven: "I am a God!" But soon this hurricane of arrogance becomes transformed. A mood of calm, muted and tranquil, takes its place; the universality of man is announced colorfully, and lighted as it were by a sulfurous dawn.

Théophile Gautier, founder with Baudelaire of the *Hachischins,* is best remembered today as a novelist, critic, and poet noted for his carefully tooled poems. His work based on the hashish experience is less remembered—possibly because his descriptions are less objective than those of Baudelaire. Gautier deals directly with the visions he encountered under the influence of the drug and does not attempt to analyze the effects. His efflorescent prose describing his intoxication was nonetheless a valuable contribution to the lore of the drug as revealed by the French *Hachischins.*

When interest in hashish lost its intellectual vogue in the second part of the nineteenth century, further accounts of the drug by European experimenters became scarce. It was not to crop up again to any significant extent until the early part of the twentieth century when sufficient evidence appears to establish the spread of the drug in Latin America and Mexico. It was to remain virtually unknown in the United States until the early twentieth century.

Why it never became popular among Europeans and Americans until recently remains a mystery. Even the hashish experiments by the members of the *Club des Hachischins* was an isolated case—the exclusive fancy of only a few intellectuals for a relatively short period of time.

If the habit of smoking cannabis began to die out in Europe toward the end of the nineteenth century, it gained rapidly in other parts of the world, despite the entangling legislation that accompanied its popularity. It is illegal in most countries, but the laws are nearly nowhere as stringent as they have been in the United States. In most places outside the U.S., with the exception of Mexico, their enforcement is seldom considered a matter serious enough to deploy the massive policing and legislative machinery found in this country.

In Algeria and other parts of North Africa and the Middle East, it is still readily available in coffeehouses; it is also widely used in Latin America where archaeological records show that marijuana and other cannabis preparations were popular before the conquest of A.D. 1509. The drug was revealed to be an important part of the religious rites of the ancient Indian empires of the Mayas and Aztecs. The reports of Spanish historians writing about the conquest of South America give evidence that a small percentage of Spaniards may also have tried the drug.

In India today, cannabis has been made illegal in many of the states but, as noted earlier, custom dictates its use among a wide percentage of the lower working classes who drink *bhang*. Whatever legal restrictions have been put into effect, the laws in most of the Indian states usually do not require the drug's concealment so that cannabis continues to be used under a much wider range of circumstances than is the case in most Western countries with similar legislation.

The use of marijuana in the United States dates back to the 1910's and 1920's, when a large influx of Mexican laborers crossed the Mexican-American border. These new arrivals coming into the Southwest brought their smoking habit with them. Having never given it much thought in their native land, they found it only natural to continue the practice in their new locations, where they planted cannabis for personal consumption. This marked its availability in this country.

"Marijuana" is somewhat of a mystery word. Its exact etymological origins have not been established, but its Mexican spelling, *marihuana,* is believed to be derived from the Mexican words for "Mary Jane." A minority opinion holds that it is a bastardization of the Portuguese word *mariguano,* meaning "intoxicant." Whatever its derivation, the term "marijuana" has been firmly established in the American drug lexicon ever since the plant was brought to this country fifty years ago.

CHAPTER TWO

THE AMERICAN EXPERIENCE: MARIJUANA IN THE UNITED STATES

From the Early Settlers to the Hippies

In the late sixteenth century, when the fleets of Europe roamed the seven seas, the Indian hemp plant was essential to European life, providing as it did the strands of flax used in the making of rope and sails for ships. Since the Dutch were in a better position to control the hemp products coming from the south of Europe, the British were forced to seek hemp products elsewhere. They decided to use the unsettled American colonies across the ocean for the production of this much-needed commodity. By the early seventeenth century, many parts of New England produced hemp, and the garments made from its fibers became so popular in America that half of the winter clothing and a good part of all summer raiment were made from it. Before long, it was necessary to step up production to supply the British fleet. James F. Hopkins, in his book *A History of the Hemp Industry in Kentucky,* reports that orders were sent from the court of King James the First of England to the new settlers to produce "iron, cordage, hemp, flax silk, pitch, tar, potash."

Studies showed that the climate and agricultural conditions of the area were ideal for the cultivation of hemp, and the year 1611 saw the first home-grown production of cannabis around Jamestown, Virginia. Although the tall gangling weed, which may reach as high as ten feet, could be seen growing in many parts of the Virginias and Kentucky, the pioneers who brought it to these states were either unaware of the effects of smoking it or refused to avail themselves of its promise of "artificial Paradise."

Hemp was also the fabric that covered the pioneers' wagons as they traveled west, and up until the time of the development of synthetic fibers, it continued to be a crop in the states of Kentucky, Virginia, Wisconsin, and Indiana, and to a lesser degree, in other states that grew cotton and corn. It is believed that George Washington raised it on his estate at Mount Vernon.

During the Colonial and post-Revolutionary periods, hemp was probably the most important southern agricultural product after cotton. Federal-government records show that before the Civil War the United States Navy awarded a contract to suppliers of Russian-grown hemp. Navy analysts favored the foreign hemp since its tensile strength was greater than that of the domestic variety, but a group of southern hemp growers pressured the government into launching a Congressional investigation of the matter.

It was finally the Industrial age and the advent of steam power in the late eighteenth century that put the hemp plantations out of business. The invention of the cotton gin at the beginning of the nineteenth century reduced the usefulness of hemp in the manufacture of textiles, and its role was subsequently limited to the production of rope.

There is, as stated earlier, no evidence that the intoxicating properties of the cannabis plant were known to the pioneers during this period in American history. The hemp was obviously planted solely for commercial purposes. It is still to be found growing either wild or cultivated in practically all of our states. Lawful cultivation is confined to the states of Kentucky, Illinois, Minnesota, and Wisconsin—where it has been estimated that, at most, ten thousand acres are devoted to legal production. Throughout the world it remains of minor commercial value in the manufacture of rope, twine, and textiles, while the seed of the plant is used as bird food. The oil extracted from the seed sometimes substitutes for linseed oil in the preparation of artists' paints.

In the United States, before the passage of the Marijuana Tax Act of 1937, hemp for ropes was mainly imported from the Far Eastern countries. During World War II, however, when these sources of supply had been cut off by Japanese occupation of the Pacific Islands, cultivation in the United States was encouraged by the federal government, which allowed special privileges and circumvention of the anti-marijuana laws. This practice was discouraged at the end of the war when the sources of foreign fiber were reopened. Later on, synthetic substitutes were developed after the war and the market for domestic hemp disappeared altogether.

The only report of early American experimentation with the drug appears in a little-known book entitled *The Hasheesh Eater: Being Passages From the Life of a Pythagorean,* published anonymously in 1860. It is now known that the author was Fitz Hugh Ludlow who lived somewhere in the neighborhood of what is now Poughkeepsie, New York.

Walking along the banks of the Hudson River, Ludlow, an intensely fanciful young man, would dream of the Orient about which he had read extensively in *Arabian Nights,* and similar books. These tales were, he says, ". . . my ceaseless marvel from earliest childhood . . . Who can rest contented with admiring the bold flights into unknown regions of imagery, and close the mystic pages that have enchanted them without an inquiry as to the influences which have turned the human mind into such rare jewels of thought?"

Arabian Nights led him to inquire into the origins of such wondrous imaginings. Reading these strange exotic tales again and again with their "strange, untrodden byways of speculation," Ludlow came to the conclusion that we in the West are unable to "account for those storm-wrapped peaks of sublimity which hover over the path of Oriental story, or those beauties which, like rivers of Paradise, make music beside it. We are all of us taught to say—'The children of the East live under a sunnier sky than their Western brethren; they are the repositors of centuries of tradition; their semi-civilized imagination is unbound by the fetters of logic and the school. . . .' "

Ludlow considered himself the first Westerner to have discovered the basis of the fantastic tales he had read as a youth. "The secret," he said, "lies in the use of hasheesh." Thus at the tender age of sixteen, the imaginative youngster began to experiment with hashish. So fascinated was he by the drug's effects on his mind that he did not end his experiments until he had left college to teach at Watertown, New York, many years later. From these early years came the material for his book.

Ludlow, it should be pointed out, admits he was strongly influenced by the Englishman Thomas De Quincey's book, *The Con-*

fessions of an Opium Eater. And when he decided to write about his experiences with the drug, the *Club des Hachischins* was flourishing three thousand miles eastward across the Atlantic Ocean on the banks of the Seine. Ludlow was probably aware of the literature produced by such members of the *Club* as Baudelaire (who had himself been influenced by De Quincey).

The American writes of his admiration for De Quincy's escape from the bonds of reality: "The path of De Quincey led beyond the boundaries of the ordinary life into a world of intense light and shadows—a realm in which all the range of average thought, found its conditions surpassed, if not violated."

Ludlow became friendly with the owner of the neighborhood apothecary from which he obtained other drugs for various experiments. In those bygone days before the creation of the Food and Drug Administration, the Narcotics Bureau, and the FBI, such pursuits were altogether legal. Ludlow could be found on many an afternoon in the apothecary's shop in Poughkeepsie sampling various potions and powders from the shelves. One morning in the spring of 1854 he dropped in upon his "favorite lounging place" to see if the pharmacist had received any new acquisitions. The apothecary pointed to the shelf bearing a row of pasteboard cylinders enclosing vials of the various extracts prepared by Tilden and Company. Ludlow took his time in examining this new shipment of drugs:

"Conium, Taraxacum, Rhubarb. . . . What is this? Cannabis Indica?"

"That," answered the doctor, "is a preparation of the East Indian hemp, a powerful agent in cases of lockjaw."

Ludlow immediately recognized the "olive-brown extract of the consistency of pitch as the hashish referred to by Eastern travelers." Placing his six cents on the counter, he took the extract with him back to his room to examine his purchase.

Ludlow first experimented with ten grains, rolled into a pill, but he experienced no effect whatsoever from this first attempt. On the following day he tried again, and continued to raise the dose by five grains each day, increasing it to twenty-five grains with still no effect. On the fifth day he was approaching the conclusion that he "was absolutely unsusceptible to the hasheesh influence." Nevertheless, he decided to give it one more try and rolled a pill of thirty grains. After supper that night he ingested the hashish. Not really expecting anything to happen, he went to the house of a friend to spend the evening. Three hours passed as he engaged in conversation with his host and listened to music, before he suddenly felt the effect of the drug take hold. He described that first experience:

> Ha! what means this sudden thrill? A shock, as of some unimagined vital force, shoots without warning through my entire frame, leaping to my finger's ends, piercing my brain, startling me till I almost spring from my chair.
>
> I could not doubt it. I was in the power of the hasheesh influence. My first emotion was one of uncontrollable terror—a sense of getting something which I had not bargained for. That moment I would have given all I had or hoped to have to be as I was three hours before. . . .
>
> Now for the first time I experienced the vast change which hasheesh makes in all measurements of time . . . with time, space also expanded . . . I was sitting at a distance of hardly three feet from the centre table around which the members of the family were grouped. Rapidly that distance widened. We were in a vast hall of which my friends and I occupied the extremities . . . I could not bear it. I should soon be left alone in the midst of infinity of space. And now more and more every moment increased the conviction that I was watched. I did not know then, as I learned afterwards, that suspicion of all earthly things and persons was characteristic of the hasheesh delirium.
>
> In the midst of my complicated hallucination, I could perceive that I had a dual existence. One part of me was whisked unresistingly along the track of this tremendous experience, the other sat looking down from a height upon its double, observing, reasoning and serenely weighing all the phenomena . . . I rose to take my leave and advanced towards the centre table. With every step its distance increased. I nerved myself as for a long pedestrian journey . . . Out in the street the view stretched endlessly away . . . I was doomed to pass through a merciless stretch of space. A soul disenthralled, setting out for his flight beyond the farthest visible star, could not be more overwhelmed with his newly acquired conception of the sublimity of distance than I was that moment. Solemnly I began my infinite journey.
>
> . . . I recognized all surrounding objects, and began calculating the distance home. Suddenly, out of a blank wall at my side a muffled figure stepped into the path before me. His hair, white as snow, hung in tangled elf-locks on his shoulders, where he carried also a heavy burden, like unto the well-filled sack of sins which Bunyan places on the back of his pilgrim. Not liking his

> manner, I stepped aside, intending to pass around him and go on my way. This change of our relative position allowed the blaze of a neighboring street-lamp to fall full on his face, which had hitherto been totally obscured. Horror unspeakable! I shall never, till the day I die, forget that face. Every lineament was stamped with the records of a life black with damning crime; it glared upon me with a ferocious wickedness and a stony despair which only he may feel who is entering on the retribution of the unpardonable sin. . . .
>
> . . . My sensations began to be terrific—not from any pain I felt, but from the tremendous mystery of all around me and within me . . . Through the thinnest corporeal tissue and the minutest veins I could trace the circulation of the blood along each inch of its progress. I knew when every valve opened and when it shut, every sense was preternaturally awakened. The beating of my heart was clearly audible. Lo, now that heart became a great fountain, whose jet played upward with loud vibrations, and, striking on the roof of my skull as on a gigantic dome, fell back with a splash and echo into its reservoir. Faster and faster came the pulsations and the stream became one continuously pouring flood, whose roar sounded through all my frame. I gave myself up for lost, since judgment, which still sat unimpaired above my perverted senses, argued that congestion must take place in a few minutes, and close the drama with my death. . . .

At this point Ludlow began to fear for his life and decided to seek medical help. The doctor he found, however, seemed to attribute his symptoms to the imagination of his patient and suggested that Ludlow go home to bed and sleep it off, which is exactly what he attempted to do. After further fantasies and visions on his way home, he finally reached his destination and jumped into bed.

The above experiences all occurred during Ludlow's first encounter with hashish. He was convinced that the Arabian and Persian storytellers were indeed influenced by the drug. Since he himself had ambitions as a writer (eventually he became a popular journalist and critic of the period), he believed that the knowledge and experience he needed could be gained from his encounters with hashish.

Accordingly, a short while after his first experience, he was off to the apothecary for another portion of the cannabis compound. He deposited his six cents on the counter and was soon back in the magic world of hashish. After a period of further experiments, he began to sum up his beliefs about the effects of hashish, spiced with generalizations about the pros and cons of the drug.

> Hasheesh I called the drug of the traveler. The whole East, from Greece to farthest China, lay within the compass of a township; no outlay was necessary for the journey. For the humble sum of six cents I might purchase an excursion ticket all over the earth.

Ludlow was to find that the destination of the hashish traveler was not always assured. The effects had very little regularity, and its actions could not be predicted.

> At two different times, when body and mind are apparently in precisely analogous states, when all circumstances, exterior and interior, do not differ tangibly in the smallest respect, the same dose of the same preparation of hasheesh will frequently produce diametrically opposite effects. Still further, I have taken at one time a pill of thirty grains, which hardly gave a perceptible phenomenon, and at another, when my dose had been half that quantity, I have suffered the agonies of a martyr or rejoined in a perfect frenzy. So exceedingly variable are its results that, long before I abandoned the indulgence, I took each successive bolus [pill] with the consciousness that I was daring an uncertainty as tremendous as the equipoise between hell and heaven. Yet the fascination employed Hope as its advocate, and won the suit.

Not infrequently the effects did plunge him into the deepest pit of hell.

> It was perhaps eight o'clock in the evening when I took the dose of fifty grains. I did not retire until midnight. I awoke suddenly. Beside my bed in the corner of the room stood a bier, from whose corners drooped the folds of a heavy pall; outstretched upon it lay in state a most fearful corpse, whose livid face was distorted with the pangs of assassination. The traces of a great agony were frozen into fixedness in the tense position of every muscle, and the nails of the dead man's fingers pierced his palms with the desperate clench of one who has yielded not without agonizing resistance . . . A smothered laugh of derision from some invisible watcher ever and anon mocked the corpse, as if triumphant demons were exulting over their prey. I pressed my hands upon my eyeballs till they ached in intensity of desire to shut out

the spectacle. I buried my head in the pillow that I might not hear that awful laugh of diabolical sarcasm.

It should be remembered that Ludlow was an extremely imaginative youth with a decided taste for metaphysical speculation. His father, an Abolitionist minister, had schooled him well in Biblical thought, the Latin and Greek classics, and as we have seen, Oriental esoterica, works that might have set his imagination aflame to the point of exaggerating the effects he experienced.

No doubt Ludlow was also guilty of incorporating some of De Quincy's agonizings over his addiction to opium. De Quincy had good reason to complain of his condition; opium addiction is definitely a serious matter, and De Quincy was an addict in the fullest sense of the word. One must, however, look with skepticism as Ludlow begins sighing and groaning over his "enslavement" to hashish. His rather theatrical breast-beating over his imaginary addiction to hashish did not last long; it appears he had little trouble discontinuing its use. Afterward, it did not seem to affect his life to any notable extent, for he never mentions any physical or mental aftereffects.

The New England teacher's experience with cannabis seems to be about the only account of this drug's usage in the United States until the early part of the twentieth century. Hashish, as opposed to marijuana—which is about a tenth as potent—never became fashionable although it was at the time legally available to anyone who could pay the price of six cents per dose. Ludlow, it should be made clear, was a lone individual who, at the time, had been influenced by the hashish users in Paris. But the public who read his book, *The Hasheesh Eater,* read it as they would one of the oriental tales that Ludlow himself read as a child—that is, as a work of pure imagination. There seemed to be no further interest on their part.

As a matter of fact, cannabis use did not achieve any great American popularity in any form whatsoever until the Mexican laborers began crossing the border, bringing with them their little bags of *mota.* There was at that time no stigma of illegality to accompany the habit. Having used marijuana in their native land, they found it natural to go on smoking it in their new country; and as they obtained jobs on ranches and orchards throughout the Southwest, they continued to plant it for personal consumption.

It should be pointed out that the type of cannabis preparation used by the Mexicans (marijuana) is a very cheap and crude preparation of the hemp plant, consisting of the tops of the female plant in all stages of development with no attempt at refinement or selection.

While the Mexican infiltration seems to have been the main influence in the adoption of the marijuana habit, there were, at the time, other groups who introduced the drug into the United States. American sailors working on ships plying between the West Indies, Central America, and the southern part of the United States also brought it in.

New Orleans, the major southern port serving these areas at the time, was the first American city to experience a marijuana cult. In the 1920's the city was a major centre for the drug and it became chic for everyone to indulge in the habit. To fulfill the demand for the weed, crops began to appear in many parts of the Southwest, but this was never to become a major source of supply because it fulfilled mainly the needs of the Mexican laborers. To satisfy the smokers in New Orleans, shipments began arriving from Havana, Tampico, and Vera Cruz, as well as from more distant parts of Mexico.

From the Gulf the marijuana habit traveled up the Mississippi via the steamboats that dispersed the goods unloaded in New Orleans. The sailors—themselves avid pot smokers—were the chief means of its distribution, and in a few short years the habit spread to every major city in the United States.

Prior to that time there had been no connection between marijuana and crime. But because the first American users were almost entirely members of underprivileged, and often disreputable, groups—Negroes, Mexican-Americans, laborers, sailors, and other members of the lower class—an arbitrary connection was made between the high crime rates in these groups and the use of marijuana. That these groups have a higher crime rate and a higher incidence of the more violent felonies whether they smoke marijuana or not was not considered. The fact that the problems of marijuana smoking frequently derive more from the kinds of people indulging in it than from the effects of the drug itself was ignored. As long as people like Ludlow, a few intellectual bohemians, some writers, doctors, scientists, and several theologians indulged primarily out of intellectual curiosity or pleasure, there did not seem to be any problem.

Similarly in France, the early experiments by a group of intellectuals with hashish produced no outcry of indignation. Neither in France nor the United States did government feel the need to pass restrictive legislation. As soon as the drug was taken up by members of a very different stratum of society, the problem began to be seen from a new viewpoint. What has since become a cultural taboo began to take shape.

The popular press of the day began to publish front-page stories of an alarmist bent about the effects of the drug on those who smoked it. There were numerous reports of users gone berserk or committing extraordinary crimes. The press whipped popular opinion to such hysteria in the early thirties that marijuana came to be automatically connected with every violent crime, especially alleged widespread corruption of school children.

Dr. R. Gomila, Commissioner of Public Safety in New Orleans in the twenties when marijuana's reputation as an evil drug first took form, wrote an article in the popular press in which he stated that some homes for boys were "full of children who had become habituated to the use of cannabis," and that "youngsters known as 'muggle-heads' fortified themselves with the narcotic and proceeded to shoot down police, bank clerks, and casual bystanders." Sixty-eight percent of the crimes committed in New Orleans in 1936 were attributed to marijuana users.

Book titles from publishers' lists at the time show a sensational slant that did little to abate popular anxiety—*Marihuana As a Developer of Criminals, Sex Crazing Drug Menace, Exposing The Marihuana Drug Evil in Swing Bands.* The newspapers continued their sensational reports. A youth in Tampa, Florida, was reported as having seized an ax and killed his father, mother, two brothers and a sister, all because he had smoked a marijuana cigarette. Armed criminals, bank robbers, kidnappers, sex maniacs, car thieves, burglars, and lawbreakers down to the lowly pickpocket, were reported to be marijuana smokers. It was not long before the newspapers and magazines came forth with an easy-reference tag for the myth they themselves had created: "The Marijuana Menace."

Across the country, organizations were set up to propagandize against its use. One of these, the Interstate Narcotic Association, mailed posters to the nation's cities to be placed "in railroad trains, buses, streetcars, etc." The wording of one of these posters, which were profusely illustrated, is indicative:

"BEWARE! Young and old people in all walks of life! This marihuana cigarette [illustration] may be handed to YOU [illustration of two clean-cut youngsters smiling innocently] by the *friendly stranger*. It contains the Killer Drug Marihuana in which lurks MURDER! INSANITY! DEATH!—WARNING! Dope Peddlers are shrewd! They may put some of this drug in the teapot [illustration] or in the cocktail or in the tobacco cigarette."

This organization informed the public that a letter "enclosing twelve cents for postage" to a given address would bring further data about the "Killer Drug." The Federal Bureau of Narcotics was "pleased with these educational campaigns describing the drug, its identification, and evil effects."

Soon other groups and individuals across the country felt called upon to combat the "evil." The Opium Advisory Association, the International Narcotic Association, and other such agencies issued masses of information that led the public to believe not only that marijuana is "a dangerous killer weed but that the majority of school children smoke the drug; that the dispensers of the drug are organized to such an extent that they encourage the use of marihuana in order to create an ever-increasing market; that juvenile delinquency is directly related to the effects of the drug; that it is the cause of a large percentage of our major crimes and sexual offenses; and that physical and mental deterioration are the direct result of the prolonged habit of smoking marihuana."

Some examples of the material issued by these organizations are enlightening. In a pamphlet entitled "Marihuana or Indian Hemp and Its Preparations" issued in 1936 by the International Narcotic Education Association, one finds a summary of the kind of information issued.

> Prolonged use of marihuana frequently develops a delirious rage which sometimes lead to high crimes, such as assault and murder. Hence marihuana has been called the "killer drug." The habitual use of this narcotic poison always causes a very marked mental deterioration and sometimes produces insanity. Hence marihuana is frequently called "loco weed." [*Loco* is the Spanish word for "crazy."]
>
> While the marihuana habit leads to physical wreckage and mental decay, its effects upon character and morality are even more devastating. The victim frequently undergoes such degeneracy that he will lie and steal without scruple; he becomes utterly

> untrustworthy and often drifts into the underworld where, with his degenerate companions, he commits high crimes and misdemeanors. Marihuana sometimes gives man the lust to kill unreasonably and without motive. Many cases of assault, rape, robbery, and murder are traced to the use of marihuana.

The alarmist newspaper reports and the propaganda produced by the various anti-marijuana organizations prompted legislators to act quickly. The main thrust behind the drive for anti-marijuana legislation was Harry J. Anslinger, the first chief of the Federal Narcotics Bureau, who remained in office until 1962. The agency enforced the laws covering the dangerous narcotics, such as heroin, opium, cocaine, and morphine, to which marijuana was added—although today there are medical authorities who do not include it in this group of narcotics but classify it as a mild hallucinogen.

The Federal Narcotics Bureau, however, identified marijuana as "a new peril—in some ways the worst we have met." It proceeded to mount an intensive campaign designed to alert the public and stimulate passage of anti-marijuana laws by all the states. The bureau worked tirelessly toward this end, and Anslinger himself appeared before a wide variety of civic organizations to speak on the subject.

The campaign was successful. In the lingering Prohibition climate of the mid-1930's, marijuana was outlawed in most states and by the federal government in 1937. Some states even surpassed the bureau's recommendations and wrote legislation into their books out of all proportion to the actual problem. The state of Oregon, for example, imposed ten-year sentences for those possessing or trafficking in the drug and many states followed suit with similar laws. Most of those state marijuana laws are more punitive than laws for armed robbery. As a matter of fact, in Georgia, sale of marijuana to a minor can mean the death penalty to an offender.

By 1936, most of the states had anti-marijuana laws and a year later the Federal Marijuana Tax Act came into being. Marijuana smokers were now, by decree, indeed criminals. Where before the argument ran that marijuana smoking produced crime, the reasoning now established that marijuana smoking *was* a crime, and the marijuana user a criminal.

The anti-marijuana legislation resulted in keeping usage predominantly among the underprivileged groups that had smoked it before the marijuana scare of the thirties. Objective knowledge about the drug remained outside the ken of the ordinary citizen. The laws that, in effect, attempted to keep smokers to a minimum or eliminate them completely, succeeded only in creating even more criminals, since those caught smoking were now automatically branded felons even if they were not involved in criminal activity. The net result was to drive the drug farther underground.

In New Orleans the police raided more than a hundred underworld dives, rounding up addicts, hardened criminals, gangsters, women of the street, sailors of all nationalities, bootleggers, muggers, and all other varieties of underworld life. Since they originally set out with a list of criminals from their own police files, it is very difficult to accept their conclusion that marijuana had led these people into a life of crime.

Official reports issued by the Commissioner of Safety of New Orleans incorporated hundreds of complaints by parents writing to the mayor as substantive evidence of the marijuana menace. They were advanced as evidence that large numbers of minors indulged in the smoking of marijuana.

Considering the sensationalism of the times, it was surprising indeed when one of New York's best-loved and most colorful mayors, Fiorello La Guardia, showed an uncommon amount of restraint and reason in dealing with the problem, especially since the New York City press had made much mileage from the new "menace." A year after the Marijuana Tax Act of 1937, popular pressure was put on the city elders to act resolutely on the tide of news reports similar to the ones published in New Orleans. As police departments rounded up thousands of suspected marijuana users as well as sellers, Mayor La Guardia sensibly concluded that his first duty was to discover the facts concerning the use of marijuana in the city before dealing with the drug. Refusing to be intimidated by the provocative newspaper reports, he appointed the world-renowned New York Academy of Medicine to make a scientific and sociological study of the use of the drug in the city of New York.

After a five-year study, the mayor's committee, appointed by the academy, produced the most exhaustive report thus far concerning marijuana and its effects. Having examined the sociological, psychological, and pharmacological aspects of the drug, the results were published in 1944 as the *Marihuana Problem in the*

City of New York—a veritable mine of valuable information. Its conclusions placed the whole phenomenon in a proper perspective.

The sociological section of the La Guardia Report showed that (1) use was predominant among Negroes, especially in the Harlem ghetto, (2) marijuana was generally smoked in the form of a cigarette, as it still is today, and (3) very few individuals ingest the weed as is common in North Africa.

The cigarettes being used at the time were rolled from three different types of tobacco. The cheapest kind of cigarettes, known as "Sass-Frass," retailed at approximately three for fifty cents (these are 1944 prices) and they were made from the less potent hemp tobacco grown in the United States. The cigarette made from tobacco grown in Mexico, Central and South America was termed the *panatella* and retailed for twenty-five cents. The strongest cigarette was *gungeon,* considered to be the highest grade of marijuana and said to be imported from Africa, although no vertification of this was available. *Gungeon* cigarettes retailed for about one dollar each.

Because of the restrictive laws, smoking of marijuana took place in Harlem "tea pads"—comfortably furnished rooms usually with a radio, phonograph, or jukebox on hand. Those who could not afford to pay the slightly higher cost of marijuana sold in the "tea pad" would usually retire to the rooftops of a building, where they smoked quietly under the stars.

Like the patron of a neighborhood tavern or bar, the marijuana smoker seemed to feel more at ease when smoking in the company of others. Again, like the social drinker, the individual in the "tea pad" seemed relaxed and freed from the anxieties that might ordinarily bother him. Unlike the often rowdy atmosphere in many lower-class bars, the "tea pads" were havens of tranquility and when, on very rare occasions, there appeared to be signs of belligerency in one of the marijuana smokers he was either ejected or forced to quiet down. The investigation revealed that there were perhaps five hundred of these "tea pads" in Manhattan.

We see from the report that the users of the 1940's continued to be members of the underprivileged classes. In the late forties, however, a new trend began to develop. Prior to that time, there had always been a sprinkling of marijuana users among the bohemian fringe of writers, intellectuals, artists, and musicians. But this group was so small in comparison to the population as a whole that it never aroused suspicion. But the period following World War II saw a decided change. Many of the young men who had fought in the war returned with more than just their battle experiences; a good number of them had sampled marijuana.

The reason for this was obvious. The military is a great social leveller, throwing together men from all classes into such close propinquity that it is only natural for them to be exposed to each other's habits. One of these habits, marijuana smoking, was to rub off on a far larger percentage of the population than would have been possible under the stricter social mores back home. Receptivity to each other's customs was not only facilitated by the chaos of war, but was transported along with footlocker and discharge papers back to the United States. Marijuana usage rapidly spread beyond the confines of the ghettos and the farm workers in the Southwest as a growing percentage of the population began to adopt this new habit.

A decade had passed since the "Marijuana Menace" scare of the thirties and, although the propaganda of the anti-marijuana groups still hung heavily in the air, the war veterans studying on the GI Bill spread its usage to campuses across America. The drug entered a whole new stratum of society. College students now encountered marijuana users of their own social class.

Another group served as a social filter for the popularization of the drug among different classes. Carrying on a musical tradition based primarily on a rural background, Negro musicians conveyed the drug experience into the jazz scene of the forties and early fifties when their music shifted to urban themes and gained a suddenly popularity with middle-class audiences. And along with the sound, their fans learned of marijuana use among the jazz musicians. The media helped to fill in the remaining lacunae in the minds of the curious.

The bohemian fringe of the day also began to emerge from the nation's woodwork into a certain measure of acceptance, if not respectability. Simultaneously, the Beat movement attracted a wide range of people from all levels of society—Negroes, college students, middle-class youths, and many of the disaffected. The central metaphor of this scene was marijuana smoking. The Beat writers—Allen Ginsberg, Jack Kerouac, William Burroughs, and many others—mentioned it more than casually in their works. The drug slowly found its level among an increasingly wider range of people.

The decade of the fifties came to be the turning point for the drug. Many Negroes were leaving the ghettos as a more distinct racial integration followed the early Civil Rights victories. What used to be the magic grass of the Negro ghetto, the jazz world, or—more recently, the hippie community—was now entering the mainstream of middle-class life.

The doctors, lawyers, executives, and housewives of today have emerged from the group of youngsters who smoked their first marijuana cigarettes during the fifties and early sixties. On many contemporary college campuses, marijuana is as much a fact of life as "frat hazings" were in the fifties. Although it is now branded as the younger generation's symbol of revolt, a "cop-out" for the disaffected, the number of serious-minded students using marijuana seems to be on the increase. Theirs is not a reaction against society at large. They smoke to escape from the academic routines, to heighten ecstatic experience, to learn more about themselves or, in some cases, simply as a social habit in the way that another generation drinks alcohol.

Although the language may be somewhat different, their gatherings do not deviate much from the standard cocktail party. Respectable types in the larger cities—lawyers, college instructors, advertising copywriters, journalists, fashion designers, artists, TV producers and writers—gather at a friend's house to smoke and socialize, to "turn on" and "drop out" temporarily from their nine-to-five world. Some individuals from a still older generation, the middle-aged doctor, businessman, corporation executive—those who did not encounter marijuana during their college years—are now crossing over to the other side of the generation gap.

The drug experience is making itself visible in all aspects of the nation's life. It is becoming increasingly apparent in television commercials, newspaper advertisements, popular films, and music. Television programs starring "hip" comics are full of overt references to grass. The old standby of the drunk act, always considered good for a few hoary laughs, has now passed out of favor. Johnny Carson's *Tonight Show* frequently makes references to the smoking of grass. And the *Jonathan Winters Show* likewise contained similar allusions to marijuana. Otto Preminger admits having smoked pot, and the world's two most celebrated ballet artists—Rudolf Nureyev and Dame Margot Fonteyn—were arrested recently for being associated with pot smokers at a party in Haight-Ashbury.

Popular music, perhaps more than any other cultural aspect, reflects the psychedelic trend. A recent song entitled "Acapulco Gold" (reputedly a high grade of marijuana) lauds the merits of pot. Teen-agers today "tune in"—if not "turn on"—to the psychedelic messages of the Beatles' "A Day in the Life" and the Rolling Stones' "Something Happened to Me Yesterday."

No one knows for certain how many Americans have tried marijuana. Former Commissioner James L. Goddard of the U.S. Food and Drug Administration was quoted by *Time* Magazine of April 19, 1968, as guessing that perhaps twenty million citizens have smoked pot at least once and that anywhere from three hundred thousand to five million smoke it regularly. Whatever the true figure, it definitely points to a permanent shift in American social habits rather than being simply a passing fad.

"The inner trip is the new response to the electric age," says "Media Master" Marshall McLuhan. "For centuries man has taken the outer trip, Columbus style. Now he has turned inward."

The most interesting development on the pot scene in the past few years has been a movement demanding not just to be able to smoke pot, but to be able to smoke pot legally. *The New Republic* has long called for the repeal of marijuana laws, adding a voice of the liberal establishment to a drive already started on college campuses and by the Beat movement. Surprisingly, *National Review,* a journal of extreme-right conservative opinion, recently published an article asking "Should We Legalize Pot?" that was answered with a resounding "Yes!" "The laws on the books today banning the sale or use of marijuana are unreasonably harsh," said Antoni Gollan, the author of the article.

In Washington, the President's Commission on Crime strongly urged that present penalties on marijuana be eased while in Great Britain the trial of the singing group, the Rolling Stones, attracted the support of such staid newspapers as *The New Statesman* and *The Spectator* to the cause of more permissive laws for marijuana. The laws dealing with marijuana, *The Spectator* states, should be "essentially legislation of control, not modeled on the legislation of prohibition."

The direction in which the "pot issue" is headed seems clear to the involved youth of today, even if it is still not so obvious to the older generation. A twenty-one-year-old student of an Ivy League College was quoted in *Newsweek* as saying that "to the new generation the future legalization of marijuana appears an inevitable result of current trends, and student leaders such as Strobe Talbott, Chairman of the *Yale Daily News,* have exhorted society to modify or repeal the existing regulations." He adds that "means of escape from the pressures of modern life are continually being devised. In America, alcohol has been the traditional after-hours lifter. Now, an additional method of diversion is being accepted—more personal and intense, perhaps, but no less valid. Even if smoking marijuana only leads to a different form of drunkenness, its legalization should be as desirable as the official sanction of alcohol. The nation is not going to flip out because I choose to smoke grass on a particular evening."

The next few years should be telling ones. The organization, LeMar, which is working for the legalization of marijuana, states that its goal should be realized by 1970 or 1971, at the latest. The group does not see any rational purpose for anti-marijuana legislation, which it believes to be an arbitrary restriction of the freedom of citizens.

It is apparent that the drug has had a rocky history in these last fifty years. Vilified and slandered at almost every turn since its emergence in New Orleans in the twenties, through the marijuana scare of the thirties, to the Negro ghettoes and migrant-labor enclaves of the forties, and from there to the campuses and Beat movement of the fifties, marijuana has come a long way to the more respectable consideration it is commanding in many quarters in the sixties.

Many physicians, however, continue to voice opposition against legalization of marijuana. Dr. Donald Louria, of New York's Cornell Medical College, was quoted in *Newsweek* of July 24, 1967, as saying: "Our society has opted for enough escape mechanisms already—liquor, caffeine and cigarettes. Why not let everyone have two barbiturates a day or two amphetamines? You have to draw the line."

Yale psychologist Kenneth Keniston sees open access to the drug as a decline in the quality of American life: "What worries me is the state of the nation where the most exciting thing available to the brightest young people is marijuana. After all, pot is a pretty poor kick, a poor substitute for real, active, exciting, meaningful experience. My complaint with marijuana is not that it hurts the smoker physically, but that it turns this bright young person away from society and robs society of his talents and energies."

The years to come will undoubtedly bring the drug's impact on our national life into sharper focus. It will be interesting to see how society reacts to such freedom if and when it becomes legal. Is the use of marijuana the "vice which draws with it a train of depravity stretching far into the future" described by Henry L. Giordano of the Bureau of Narcotics? Or, is its indulgence "something that is sometimes right and sometimes wrong, without hard and fast rules . . . a question left up to the individual," as maintained by Northwestern University sociologist Howard Becker when he studied the pot culture in the fifties? The verdict will depend largely on the outcome of the cross-country challenge to present federal and state marijuana laws.

CHAPTER THREE

WHAT IS POT? THE MARIJUANA PLANT

Cannabis Sativa and Mary Jane

What exactly is pot? Or tea, or grass, or hay, or gage, or charge, or boo, or woolie, or green? They all refer to marijuana as do literally hundreds of other slang terms for the drug—some that are known to millions, and others, to only a small coterie or minority group. Like slang in general, these words serve as a shield against the prying eyes of the "square" world. They apply either to the plant itself or to various preparations made from its leaves or resins.

The marijuana plant, which grows to a height of anywhere between five to ten feet, looks like a large weed and most resembles a scrawny nettle. Although originally indigenous to Central Asia, Indian hemp is now found in practically every section of the world.

In 1752 the eighteenth-century scientist Linnaeus described the plant with some scientific accuracy, christening the species *Cannabis sativa.* Today's botanists call it *Cannabis sativa L.* But even before that the Greeks had a word for it, as did the Persians, Arabs, Africans, Hindus, Chinese, and Indians. No matter what the terminology, all the terms apply to a single species of plant—the tall, weedy annual herb related to the fig tree and the hop, and a distant relation to the stinging nettle.

There is still some disagreement over the proper classification of the plant. One group of botanists place it in the mulberry family, while others include it in a group that covers the hop plant. (Hops produce a special resin from which beer gets its bitterness, its aroma, and its slightly soporific qualities; similarly, the potent spirit of hemp also resides in a sticky and aromatic resin that coats the female flowers of the plant.)

The marijuana plant has a hollow, herbaceous, and four-cornered stalk that at maturity may reach a two-inch diameter. In the proper climate it can far surpass its average height of five to ten feet and reach up to twenty feet. Depending on the location of the plant, the leaves will usually continue to sprout while the branches spread to widths of five to ten feet. The leaves are long, approximately five to ten inches; five to eight leaves usually sprout from one bud on the branch. In appearance the leaves are dark green, pointed at both ends and serrate.

Modern botanists know that *Cannabis sativa* grows in two forms. One is the tall and comparatively colorless male plant, the stem of which yields a cordage fiber known as hemp. The female, although shorter, is the more interesting one since it is the producer of the cannabis drug. In their early stages, the male and female plants are similar in most respects but, as they grow to full height, the differences become apparent. As the maturing process unfolds, the male plant blossoms, spreads its pollen to the female plant, and then dies. The male plant, however, is useless for smoking because it produces only very minute amounts of the resin that contains the intoxicating quality of the drug.

On the other hand, the female plant develops a sticky protective coating that gathers on and around its upper reproductive parts. This coating is developed as protection and insulation during the reanimative process. The resin keeps the reproductive parts of the female plant moist and prevents evaporation from this area. In an extremely moist climate, production of this resin is unnecessary and the plant will therefore have little value if collected for intoxicating purposes. Dry climates, such as are found in North Africa and parts of India, produce a protective coating that is extremely generous. The air in certain parts outside Bombay, India, has a soporific quality that would be familiar to anyone who has ever been around hop fields at harvest time. Just as the hop resin is used for giving beer its body, the intoxicating resin of the female hemp plant is the potent ingredient in the making of the various cannabis preparations.

Depending on the end product desired, cultivators of the Indian hemp plant use various methods in harvesting it. In the sections of India that produce cordage, since the stem of the male plant yields a better fiber for hemp-rope production than the female, most of the female plants are destroyed except for a small number required to produce the seed needed for the next planting. Where the intoxicating resin is desired, such as in parts of North Africa, the male plant is destroyed after it has matured and pollinated the female.

Depending on the environment, the life span of the Indian hemp plant varies from three months to one year. Since the plant is an extremely hardy weed it will reproduce itself naturally by its own seed. However, it is usually seeded by farmers raising it for cultivation purposes.

In the United States, where cultivation is illegal with the exception of just a few states, a more haphazard method is used. Seeds may be sprinkled in an empty field and the mature product reaped later. The illegal cultivator will be careful not to tend the plants before reaping because of the chance of arrest. His activities are further hampered by the fact that the plant will not thrive in a shaded area. The open, sunny field in which it must be raised makes it difficult to conceal illegal cultivation.

In the larger cities, urban entrepreneurs favor vacant lots, abandoned construction sites, secluded backyards, and the rooftops of apartment buildings for their home-grown marijuana. Cultivation is made easier by reason of the fact that Indian hemp will thrive in practically any type of soil.

A recent Federal Bureau of Narcotics raid in New York City discovered a major crop growing in the basement of a huge apartment complex. The superintendent of the building had strung up dozens of sun lamps to shine on the seeds he had planted in the soil of the cellar's dirt floor. The *Marijuana Newsletter*, an underground hippie newspaper, facetiously described a marijuana offshoot that grows in the sewers of Manhattan, Manhattan Silver. "It originated when potheads began flushing seeds down their toilets during police raids. It grows without benefit of sunlight. It varies in color from white to silver and it is the strongest grade on the market."

The conditions under which the plant is raised affect the potency of the final product. As the La Guardia Report stated some years back, this was noticeable by even the smokers of the relatively mild marijuana preparation. The minimum of attention given to crops raised in the United States makes it the poorest in quality. Next comes the marijuana imported from Mexico, Central and South America where the indigenous people are not as cognizant of the care required in cultivating the hemp crop as are those in Africa and India who have known it for thousands of years. The best supply comes specifically from the Middle East, North and West Africa, Northwest India—especially the area north of Bombay—and more recently, the West Indies where cultivators have been quick to adapt themselves to the demands of a lucrative market.

Because hemp seeds remain fertile for only a few years, it is necessary to keep a small crop on hand in case an emergency such as war makes it necessary to raise hemp once again for the production of rope. The United States Department of Agriculture as well as the Bureau of Narcotics keep a close eye on the possible illicit cultivation of the plant. A recent warning issued to farmers in the *Farmers' Bulletin* reads: "Warning: The hemp plant contains the drug marijuana. Any farmer planning to grow hemp must comply with certain regulations of the Marijuana Tax Act of 1937. This involves registration with the farmer's nearest Internal Revenue Collector and the payment of a fee of one dollar. Although the fee is small, the registration is mandatory and should not be neglected, as the penalty provision for not complying with the regulation is very severe."

Despite the obstacles put in its way, the Indian hemp plant continues to flourish as it has for more than five thousand years. The resin that has caused concern to some and pleasure to others ever since an inquisitive native first discovered its extraordinary properties continues to be gathered from the plant's flowering top. Since the cannabis drug derives its potency from the resin of the flowering tops of the female Indian hemp plant, various preparations are used around the world.

Marijuana is the most common preparation of the cannabis drug used in North America. The variety grown in America is influenced by location, soil, and weather conditions; nevertheless, it is basically the same plant, with a resin identical to that produced by plants grown in Asia and Africa, although the preparation may not be as potent.

The resin as the active intoxicating principle may be ingested or inhaled after being prepared in various ways, but marijuana virtually always comes in the form of tobacco and is invariably smoked, especially in North America.

Marihuana, the Mexican name for the North American preparation, supposedly referred to a cheap type of ordinary Mexican tobacco, "Mary Jane," which subsequently lent its name to the intoxicating cannabis. Aside from the vernacular of the streets, *marihuana* is the only term used for this preparation in North America. Contemporary terms to distinguish the various qualities of the drug seem to be chiefly apocryphal, since it is near impossible to trace the various brand names to the location in which they are presumed to be grown. Acapulco Gold, Panama Red, Quintana Roo Blue are a few of the terms experienced potheads use to differentiate between the varieties of marijuana.

The preparation of marijuana is absurdly easy; it simply involves mashing the dried and crumpled leaves, stems, and seeds. A more potent product results from using only the leaves and stem of the upper part of the plant, which has a higher concentration of resin. Pure marijuana is a blend of ripe hemp leaves, some of which may have lots of resin, while others contain very little or none at all. Sometimes the marijuana imported from Mexico is mixed with ordinary tobacco in the United States before being distributed. When this happens, it may be inferred that the Mexican marijuana was of extraordinary strength, making a smaller amount both more valuable and easier to conceal in crossing the border. In these cases it is likely that only the top portion of the mature plant was used.

Bhang is the Indian equivalent of marijuana. This preparation is similarly derived from the leaves, stem, and stalks of the female Indian hemp plant. Since the quality depends on that portion of the plant with the strongest resin contents, its Indian derivation from mainly uncultivated plants lowers the potency considerably. Sometimes the complete plant is dried and ground up as is done with marijuana, but more usually the uncultivated backyard plants are simply cut up to be brewed in a decoction of milk or water. The liquid is then drunk like coffee or tea. *Bhang,* probably the cheapest way to obtain the cannabis drug, is used mainly among the very poor in India. The *kif* of the Middle East and the *dagga* of Africa are both prepared in a roughly similar manner and have about the same potency.

Ganja is still another preparation from India, approximately two to four times as potent as either marijuana or *bhang.* This variety of hemp is also usually selected from Indian hemp plants specifically cultivated for this purpose. The plant not only grows better in the hot climate of India (hotter than the United States or Mexico), but it is also given far greater care while being cultivated. Instead of using the complete plant as is usually the case with marijuana, great selectivity is employed in picking only the finest tops of the healthiest female plants. Since the tops are carefully cut before being used in the various smoking mixtures, this method allows for a greater concentration of resin than is found in marijuana.

In India *ganja* is smoked by those who can afford to pay more than they would for the cheaper-grade *bhang*. Like *bhang,* it is sometimes brewed in water or milk but it is more generally smoked. As a liquid solution, *ganja* is favored in the West Indies, where it is prized for its therapeutic efficacy in connection with voodoo rites. The high priest administers the potation to the celebrants in a soul-cleansing ritual that, according to witnesses, is similar in its effects to the results wrought by Bible-thumping faith healers in the United States. *Ganja* is also used in feminine sweetmeats similar to the Middle Eastern *majum*.

Made from the same carefully cultivated plants that go into the production of *ganja,* the Indian *charas* comes from the finest tops of the finest plants. It is in fact the pure, unadulterated resin from the highest-quality Indian hemp. Unlike *ganja,* which mixes other parts of the plant together with the resin, *charas* only contains the pure resin distilled from the sticky flowers. This resin is either dried and crushed into a powder, or made into small cakes that look rather like boullion cubes. These blocks may subsequently be crumbled into powder and mixed with tobacco to be smoked. They may also be smoked in small lumps through a special pipe or as an additive to various other preparations. This almost pure substance is approximately five to ten times as potent as marijuana or *bhang*.

The proper preparation and cultivation of *charas* is best accomplished in India, where special skills have been developed over the years to promote the secretion of the intoxicating resin. The ancient custom in collecting the first secretions of the resin was to send naked men running with outstretched arms through rows of hemp. At the end of such a run, the sticky substance adhering to their skin was then scraped off. Today the cut flower clusters are spread between white cheesecloth. This is pressed to coax out the resin, which is then scraped from the surface of the cloth.

The preparation of *charas,* the nearly pure resin of the hemp plant and flowers, spread to North Africa where it has been known as *hasheesh* ever since the days of Hasan and his band of "assassins." Today *hasheesh* is the more popular name for this preparation in the Middle East although it goes back many hundreds of years before it gained its North African nomenclature. Although the relation between marijuana and hashish is comparable to that between beer and pure alcohol, hashish is equivalent to marijuana in its chemical composition and psychological effects. The only difference is that a lesser amount of hashish achieves the same effects as those of marijuana.

Although an Israeli scientist recently claimed to have isolated the intoxicant in the cannabis resin, its synthesization is hampered by the difficulty in locating its specific active ingredients. The first two substances to be isolated were cannabinol and cannabidiol. The latter compound is considered the more relevant of the two in producing the intoxicating quality.

Another closely related compound, tetrahydrocannabinol (THC), seems to be the closest the chemists have come to producing the active ingredients by synthesis. THC has been extracted not only from the hemp resin, but it was also created synthetically and semisynthetically. It has never been isolated from cannabis in a homogeneous crystalline form.

THC does not seem to exhibit an exact parallel to the effects of the cannabis drug. Investigations carried out independently in Czechoslovakia and Germany between the years 1955 to 1960 have shown that, besides THC, there are other components in the cannabis drug with different biological properties. The recently isolated cannabidiolic acid was found to be a sedative and antibacterial agent of this drug. Numerous studies carried out in Canada, Poland, Germany, Italy, Czechoslovakia, the United States, and Yugoslavia employed new analytical methods to probe the chemical storehouse of cannabinol as well as other constituents of cannabis.

As the main biological agent, THC remains the center of interest in the study to identify the chemical reactions taking place in the cannabis drug. The THC's themselves are easily synthesized, regardless of their exact relationship to the cannabis drug, and they do produce a similar intoxication. Although a "marijuana pill" has been produced from the THC's, this product has failed to make a stir among pot enthusiasts.

As the La Guardia Report on marijuana has shown, smoking rather than ingesting a pill seems to be the preferable method, allowing control over the intoxication, and therefore, a more satisfying experience for the smoker. Puffing at a "joint" certainly exerts a measure of control over intake of the drug, enabling the user to calculate the progressive stages of his "high." The La Guardia Report also pointed out that the smoker of marijuana usually will smoke only so much of the drug for fear of shattering his high.

Another synthetic that approximates the active principles of marijuana is synhexyl. It was discovered by Dr. Roger Adams who isolated and synthesized a number of the chemical properties of marijuana. Synhexyl was tested at the Federal Hospital in Lexington, Kentucky (an institution for the cure of narcotics addicts), where it was used as a therapeutic device, particularly as a euphoriant for the depressive mental states produced by withdrawal from the hard narcotics. It was discovered, however, that this drug also fails to produce the exact effects of marijuana. The pharmacological properties of synhexyl, although in many ways similar to those of the cannabis drug, exhibit several important qualitative differences in the human system. Synhexyl is more potent weight for weight than is natural cannabis, the effective dosage being five to fifteen milligrams in the normal subject.

In addition, the effects of synhexyl take twice as long in coming as those of cannabis, and when the high does arrive, it is rather sudden compared to the more gradual effects of its natural counterpart. Further, no hallucinatory phenomena have been encountered with synhexyl as is sometimes the case with cannabis.

Before anyone can be incriminated under the Marijuana Tax Law of 1937, the drug must be definitely identified as marijuana. Since the law relates marijuana to any part of the *Cannabis sativa* plant, a botanist is usually employed to finger and compare the tobacco to the standard means of identification. This is done mainly by examining the underside of the leaf, which is rather unique because its veins trace a definite pattern while the serrated edge presents another clearly distinctive characteristic. Color, texture, and seeds are other facets of the identification process, although the most important incriminating evidence continues to be the cystolith hair of the leaf. If the leaves have not been crushed to a powder, the matter is relatively simple.

The chemical or Duquenois test is used by the Bureau of Narcotics when the more obvious properties of the plant have been destroyed. In this assay a chemical is added to the material, producing a color change that verifies the presence of the cannabis ingredient.

The legal classification of marijuana is not so simple. According to the medical evidence presently available, it is still on rather shaky ground. Marijuana has been ranked as a narcotic along with the hard drugs, heroin, cocaine, and morphine, although scientific evidence fails to completely support this classification. Most medical experts agree that, unlike heroin and morphine, marijuana does not result in physical addiction. Unlike the narcotics user, the cannabis smoker does not develop a tolerance to marijuana and has no need for ever-increasing doses to obtain satisfaction.

The La Guardia Report has demonstrated that the user deprived of marijuana does not suffer the intense craving, chills, and nausea typical of withdrawal of the hard narcotics. Most pharmacologists today would place marijuana in a classification with the other hallucinogens, LSD, peyote, etc.

Meanwhile, the hardy marijuana plant continues to thrive, practically in the midst of all the controversy. In North America, the plant grows wild in the southern United States, a roadside weed. The Mexican farmer simply drops seeds into holes in the ground, tramples them down with his feet, and never gives them another thought until he returns for the harvest from four to seven months later. Even urban afficionados can sometimes surreptitiously raise a small backyard crop.

In this respect, nature seems to be on the side of the pot smokers.

CHAPTER FOUR

WHAT POT DOES: THE PHARMACOLOGY OF MARIJUANA

Its Physical and Psychic Effects

The reports of Baudelaire, Gautier, and Ludlow provided Europe and America with their first inkling of the mind-altering compounds found in nature's pharmacopoeia. Although the effects described are relatively accurate, they are literary effusions and metaphysical speculations far removed from the scientific objectivity with which the drug must be examined if its true nature is to be revealed.

Up until 1937, when marijuana was outlawed in this country, some research was still taking place but it was largely discontinued after the drug became increasingly difficult to obtain. With the scare campaign that preceded and followed the passing of the Marijuana Tax Act, smaller and larger misconceptions have helped to obscure its true nature up until this day. It was even dropped from the official *United States Pharmacopoeia* after passage of the restrictive legislation. In the United States, marijuana became almost more fabled than the hashish of *Arabian Nights.*

What exactly are the effects of marijuana? How extensive is our popular knowledge of marijuana? And how accurate is this knowledge?

Fortunately, a number of studies testing the drug have been made. Until quite recently the La Guardia Report was the only thorough body of work on the subject, but late in 1968 it was joined by a new study completed at the Boston University Medical Center, which published its findings in December of that year.

Its overall report will be examined later in this chapter. Meanwhile, let us first turn to the earliest report on record.

The *Report of the Indian Hemp Drug Commission,* a marijuana study published in 1894, was an inquiry that comprised more than three thousand pages, and took nearly two years to complete. It was conducted with typical British impartiality while the Union Jack still flew over India. The commission interviewed hundreds of Indians from all social classes—coolies and fakirs, physicians and marijuana dealers, Army officers and the clergy. After an exhaustive examination of every possible aspect of cannabis use in India, from the production of the drug to the various houses in which the drug was smoked, it came to the conclusion "that the drug does not result in any mental or moral injuries or cause disease."

Although quite a few scientific studies have been carried out in India and the Middle East, they have been concerned primarily with *hasheesh, kif,* and *ganja,* and other forms of the cannabis drug that are more powerful than the marijuana found in North America. The immediate need called for a source of information that would be compiled by trained scientific investigators. The first such objective study, hedged by numerous scientific controls, was that carried out by Mayor La Guardia's Committee on Marijuana. Its opus, published in 1944, *The Marihuana Problem in the City of New York,* commonly referred to as the La Guardia Report, contains sociological, clinical, and pharmacological reports that are probably the best available on the subject. An amazingly thorough and well-documented volume, its findings are extremely relevant to the current debate.

When petitioned by Mayor La Guardia, the renowned New York Academy of Medicine's Committee on Public Health Relations appointed a special scientific team (the Mayor's committee) consisting of thirty-two eminent physicians, psychiatrists, clinical psychologists, pharmacologists, chemists, and sociologists. They were charged with the task of conducting a painstaking two-part inquiry—a sociological study to evaluate marijuana use in the community, and a clinical study to evaluate the drug's effects under laboratory conditions.

The entire medical staff of New York's Prison Hospital on Riker's Island, two wards of Goldwater Memorial Hospital, a staffed laboratory to conduct experiments, and the Department of Pharmacology of Cornell Medical School headed by Dr. S.

Lowe were pressed into the service of the investigating team. The result was a report that, although issued a good twenty-five years ago, is still the most impressive collection of factual findings in the whole body of scientific literature on marijuana. As Mayor La Guardia himself acknowledged, "The report of the present investigations covers every phase of the problem and is of practical value, not only to our own city, but to communities throughout the country. It is a basic contribution to medicine and pharmacology."

Our concern in this chapter will be mainly with the clinical study that sought "to determine by means of controlled experiment (involving seventy-two prisoner-volunteers) the physiological and psychological effects of marijuana on different kinds of persons; the question as to whether it causes physical or mental deterioration; and its possible therapeutic effects on the treatment of disease or other drug addiction."

The marijuana used by the researchers was in the form of an alcohol fluid concentrate of the active principle of the cannabis drug (an oral form supplied by the Consulting Chemist of the United States Treasury Department) and marijuana cigarettes (obtained from supplies confiscated by the New York City Police Department). The part of the clinical study contained in the La Guardia Report that interests us here are the sections covering the medical aspects (symptoms and behavior, and the organic and systemic functions); the psychological aspects (the psychophysical and other functions, intellectual functioning, and emotional reactions and general personality structure); and comparisons between users and nonusers from the standpoint of mental and physical deterioration.

When smoked, the marijuana drug quickly passes into the bloodstream, reaching the brain center in a matter of minutes. The oral dose administered by the La Guardia research group took a little longer in showing its effects. Since the appointed task force wanted to give a completely detached and scientific viewpoint, they discarded the information contained in the literature then available on the subject. Instead, five volunteers were engaged in a preliminary study to set up a system of procedures that could be employed in experiments with the main group to follow later.

The first general symptoms noted after administering an oral dose to these subjects were a slight increase in pulse rate and blood pressure, dilated and sluggish pupils, dryness of the mouth and throat, ataxia, and some clumsiness and incoordination of movement. Among the disagreeable symptoms observed were dizziness, a heavy sensation in the extremities, nausea, faintness, and some restlessness. Laughter, witticism, loquaciousness, and lowering of inhibitions occurred in most subjects, although there was also evidence of difficulty in sustaining mental concentration and spells of disagreeable symptoms. Sexual stimulation was never apparent and the overall effects of the oral dose usually lasted between two and four hours. The effects of smoking the drug ranged from one to three hours.

The medical team then went on to study the main group of volunteers using both the oral concentrate and marijuana cigarettes, where they found results similar to the ones observed in the preliminary group. Although not true in all cases, the duration of the action and intensity of the marijuana tended to increase with dosage. The reason for occasional variances in the general pattern was explained by "differences in the mental makeup of the subjects, and the particular state of mind and responsiveness at the time the marihuana is taken"—in other words, the "set" of the subject as Timothy Leary has defined it for the LSD experience. The results showed that specific effects varied with the individual, some of whom remained quiet, showing little interest in their surroundings, while others were restless and talkative.

Euphoria occurred in one form or another in most of the subjects. These were "a sense of well-being and contentment, cheerfulness and gaiety, talkativeness, bursts of singing and dancing, daydreaming, a pleasant drowsiness, joking and performing amusing antics. The drowsiness, daydreaming, and unawareness of surroundings were present when the subject was left alone. Other euphoric expressions required an audience and there was much contagiousness of laughing and joking where several of the subjects under marihuana congregated. The occurrence of a euphoric state in one form or another, was noted in most of the subjects."

Difficulty in focusing and sustaining mental concentration showed themselves in the subjects as a delay in answering questions put to them and some confusion as to their meaning. There was, however, "no abnormal mental content evident and responses brought out by the examiner were not different from those in the pre-marihuana state."

The symptoms of "a feeling described as lightness, heaviness or pressure in the head, often with dizziness occurred in practically all subjects." About half of them reported a dryness of the mouth and a floating sensation, unsteadiness of movement, and a feeling of heaviness in the extremities. Hunger pangs and a desire for sweets were commonly experienced. Present, but less common were "nausea, vomiting, sensations of warmth of the head or body, burning of the eyes, and blurring of vision, tightness of the chest, cardiac palpitation, ringing or pressure in the ears, and an urge to urinate or defecate." Tremor and ataxia were present in varying degrees, as well as dilation of the pupils and sluggish response to light.

The actions of marijuana as exhibited in symptoms and behavior were found to last from two to three hours and never longer than five hours.

Left undisturbed, this group displayed some difficulty in sustaining mental concentration and seemed unaware of their physical surroundings. In company, though, they were restless, talkative, laughing, and joking. Apprehension, when it occurred, involved uncertainty about the effects of the drug. This was increased by any disagreeable sensations present, although it was never expressed in violent or aggressive ways.

A transfer of the catalog of symptoms to smokers placed in less clinical surroundings easily yields a picture of the marijuana user in society. One of the symptoms observed was a dryness of the mouth and a craving for food, especially sweets. Just as the hostess of a cocktail party sets out a tray of snacks, the pot party usually sports a supply of soft drinks, coffee, tea, soup, cocoa, lemonade, or any other likely beverage. Alcoholic beverages are rare since they tend to reduce the effects of marijuana. Because of the American sweet tooth, soda pop is most favored at such get-togethers.

Such possible physical effects as unsteadiness, sensations of heaviness in the extremities, and clumsiness of movement will usually keep the smoker in situations that require little or no physical effort. He prefers to engage in conversation, listen to music, or watch television. These behavior symptoms are in direct contrast to those produced by alcohol, which usually induce overt expression of the released inhibitions, as opposed to the turning inward of the marijuana smoker.

The La Guardia group also studied the functions of the body organs and systems under the influence of the cannabis drug to ascertain "whether subjects who had long been using the drug gave evidence of organic damage." Tests were made before, during, and after administering marijuana. The medical experts paid special attention to the functioning of the heart and circulation, blood composition, kidney, liver and gastro-intestinal function, and basal metabolism.

They observed an increase in the pulse rate, which reached its peak in about two hours, as marijuana's most consistent effect. Although it gradually dropped after hitting its peak, the increased pulse rate was usually accompanied by a rise in blood pressure. A slight rise in the blood-sugar level and in the basal-metabolic rate, as well as a frequent need to urinate, were not considered to exceed the normal level. The craving for candy and soda pop was observed to have an interesting side effect in preventing the subject from getting too high. Additionally, there were no appreciable differences in the composition of the blood and the circulation rate from the pre-marijuana state, while the electrocardiogram showed no abnormal departures caused by the drug.

Positive note was taken of the fact that the effects recorded were not intensified by an increased dosage. The preceding reactions to the drug were also explained as expressions of forms of cerebral excitation that had no direct relation to the action of the drug on any of the organs observed. Marijuana was said to act upon the central nervous system, which in turn affected the organs.

A number of tests run to determine the effects of marijuana on various psychomotor and mental abilities included some novel experiments. The functions tested were (1) static equilibrium (measured by means of the Miles ataximeter, an instrument for recording body sway); (2) hand steadiness (measured by means of the Whipple steadiness tester, which consists of a mental disc with a hole and a stylus); (3) speed of tapping (measured by the Whipple apparatus in somewhat the same manner as hand steadiness); (4) strength of grip (using the Collins dynamometer); (5) simple and complex hand-and-foot reaction time (for which a special apparatus was constructed); (6) musical aptitude (determined by means of the Kwalwasser-Dykema music tests, covering tonal memory and movement, discrimination of quality, intensity, time, rhythm, and pitch, and melodic taste); (7) auditory acuity (tested by means of the Galton whistle); (8) perception of time (where the subject indicates the intervals elapsed after a certain signal); and (9) perception of length (where the subject was asked to estimate the length of lines shown him).

The volunteers took these tests before smoking marijuana; a week later under the influence of two cubic centimeters and finally, after the elapse of another week with five cc. of the drug.

The complexity of the function tested was found to be the chief factor in determining psychomotor reactions to the drug. The simpler functions (such as tapping) showed little or no evidence of being affected by marijuana. Even larger doses affected them only slightly. Regardless of large or small doses, more complex functions, such as static equilibrium, were hampered considerably after administration of the drug. Body and hand steadiness were particularly affected, especially in volunteers who had never used the drug before.

Marijuana failed to produce an adverse reaction in either auditory acuity or sense of time and linear distance, nor was there any evidence that the drug—among the nonmusicians tested—improved musical ability, although the subjects did express greater appreciation for the music played in other experiments.

The tests used in determining marijuana's effect on the intellectual process included (1) the Wechsler adult-intelligence test (to measure the general mental level of all subjects); (2) the Army alpha test (a group of tests first employed in the United States Army); (3) Pyle's digit-symbol test (in which the learning rate is recorded by how fast the subject can associate the numbers 1 through 9 with specific symbol); (4) the cancellation test (to measure the individual's capacity for carrying out a routine task); (5) the Forum board test (to determine the ability to manipulate concrete material in contrast to verbal or abstract ability); (6) the Kohs block design test (a board test independent of language but relying on abstract intelligence); and (7) the memory test (the ability to recall presented objects and visual memory).

Administered in either pill or cigarette form, the marijuana generally had an adverse effect on the subject's mental processes, although this result was always transitory. The dosage played a major role in the extent and duration of the intellectual impairment, with smaller doses producing the least disturbance. Again, as with the effects on the psychomotor functions, the complexity of the function tested determined the extent of the intellectual deterioration. The more involved the function, the more severely it was affected by the drug.

Nonusers of marijuana were found to experience greater loss of intellectual ability, and for longer periods, than the experienced marijuana smokers. The loss of both speed and accuracy caused by the drug were held responsible for its effects on the intellectual functioning of the subject. They were not permanent, however, lasting only for the duration of the experiment, and the researchers found in long-range testing that "indulgence in marijuana does not appear to result in mental deterioration."

In order to determine the changes in emotional reaction and general personality structure, a number of tests were given, to both the marijuana user and nonuser. The tests employed were: (1) the Rorschach test (an analysis of personality by means of responses to ink blots and drawings); (2) the Goodenough test (personality diagnosis by means of a figure of a man drawn by the subject); (3) level-of-aspiration test (determination of the relationship between the goal a person sets for himself and the level of his performance); (4) the frustration test (in which the subject's frustration is observed in his accomplishment of a task); (5) the Binet line-suggestibility test (in which the subject's response to suggestibility is observed); (6) the Wechsler vocational interest test (analysis of the subject's personality from his choice of job preference); (7) the Loof-Bourrow personal-index test (to measure proneness to deliquency); (8) the Wechsler free-association test (a word test used in personality study); (9) the Pressey X-O test (another word test for personality study); (10) the thematic apperception test (in which the needs of the subject are revealed in his stories and the environmental forces acting upon him); and (11) the Downey will-and-temperament test (to determine personality traits).

This last test was highly relevant for it was used in this study solely to determine if marijuana produces changes in the individual's self-evaluation—and, if so, what kinds of changes. By comparing the traits that the individual under normal circumstances thinks apply to him, and the traits he thinks apply to him when he is under the influence of marijuana, the researchers could reach conclusions as to the drug's supposed anti-Establishment and crime-inducing properties.

The testing of the subjects in both the drugged and undrugged experiments were as widely spaced in time as possible. The general conclusion reached by the La Guardia researchers for all the above tests was that "under the influence of marihuana changes in personality as shown by alteration of test performance are slight. They are not statistically significant."

Conclusive evidence shows the personality changes that did occur were demonstrated in a reduction in drive, less objectivity in evaluating situations, less aggression, and a generally more favorable attitude toward the subject himself. These, the report added, were the result of two main causes—an increased feeling of relaxation and disinhibition as well as increased self-confidence The effect of the drug loosened the restraint the subject normally imposed upon himself and he spoke more freely than he would in the undrugged state. "Metaphysical problems, which in the undrugged state the subject would be unwilling to discuss, sexual ideas he would ordinarily hesitate to mention, jokes without point, are all part of the oral stream released by the marihuana."

The study also found that there was a reduction in the individual's critical faculty, due probably to the intellectual confusion produced by the drug's relaxing influence. Some lack of drive to achieve the goals considered worthwhile in the undrugged state was another trait evinced by the subject after smoking marijuana. In other physical areas the subject reported a pleasant drifting and floating sensation without any feelings of pressure or compulsion to do anything in particular.

In the administration of larger doses of the drug—five cc. as compared with two taken orally—feelings of anxiety, and in some cases, of physical distress, such as nausea, overcame the pleasurable sensations. The subject's confidence was eroded until feelings of insecurity became pronounced enough to evoke generally negativistic attitudes to most of the stimuli.

Smoking marijuana, rather than oral ingestion, it was found, was a more effective regulator of the dosage sufficient to bring on the high and usually prevented the type of overindulgence that caused the feelings of anxiety. The smaller dose (2 cc.) appeared to be the amount the subject would take if left to his own devices.

One of the most important findings of the La Guardia Report was the fact that the drug does not affect the basic outlook of the individual except in a very few instances and then to a very slight degree. In general, the subjects who are withdrawn and introspective stay that way, those who are outgoing remain so, and so on. Where changes occur, the shift is so slight as to be negligible. In other words, reactions that are natively alien to the individual cannot be induced by the ingestion or smoking of the drug.

In summing up marijuana's influence on the emotional reactions and general-personality structure, the La Guardia Report concluded that: (1) the individual's basic personality structure does not change except for a few superficial alterations; (2) the individual experiences increased feelings of relaxation, disinhibition, and self-confidence; (3) these new feelings of self-confidence express themselves primarily through verbal rather than physical activity, which is generally diminished; (4) the disinhibition resulting from the use of marijuana releases the individual's basic personality characteristics, but does not cause him to react in ways alien to him; (5) feelings of anxiety may frequently be released; (6) individuals who have difficulty in making social contacts are more likely to resort to marijuana than their more extroverted counterparts.

It readily follows that marijuana cannot be the cause of criminal tendencies since the drug does not affect the smoker's basic personality structure. It has been shown that unlike alcohol, which seems to induce feats of daring, marijuana increases the feeling of relaxation and tends to decrease physical activity. Since the drug tends to aid the introvert in relating to his environment, it would seem that those who are disaffected with society—the withdrawn and alienated—are the ones most drawn to the drug.

The percentage of criminals from such a group would show a natural tendency to be larger than that of an average cross-section of society. Despite this, the report found that the criminals who used marijuana tended to limit their activities to the more petty crimes of picking pockets, breaking and entering, and the like. Although very few violent crimes were reported in connection with marijuana smokers, it should be kept in mind that these findings held true for the situation as it existed when marijuana was used mainly by the alienated minority groups of the ghettoes, where the crime rate was higher than the national average. Today, with many college students having tried the drug and a good percentage continuing to use it, it would only follow that if the alarmist theories were correct, the country would now be awash under a flood of criminals pouring out of the halls of academe across the nation.

Since the active principles of marijuana have not yet been identified, its biological activities are a mosaic of uncertain compositions. Much work in uncovering the drug's secrets still remains to be done.

"In all probability the chemical constitution of this unique substance is not going to be definitely recognized until there is a coordinated investigative program in which the chemical alterations are guided directly by accurate measurements of physiological activity." This from Dr. R. P. Walton's *Marijuana: America's New Drug Problem* (published by J. B. Lippincott Company, Philadelphia, Pa.), which reviews the period of unsuccessful endeavor to isolate the active principles of marijuana, adequately sums up the prevailing scientific view on the subject.

The La Guardia study also attempted to track down marijuana's active principle in a series of experiments at the Cornell University Medical College. They knew that the drug affected the higher cerebral functions, including its psychic actions, producing euphoria and relaxation. Its effects, grouped under the heading "Marihuana Activity" were found to reside in all of the numerous preparations obtained from members of the *Cannabinaceae* family. Despite minor differences in the various plant species and nomenclature throughout the world (*Cannabis Americana,* in the United States of America and Mexico; *Cannabis Indica* in India; *Cannabis Sinensis,* in China; etc.), they all belong to the same family.

The resin was examined to see which part of the plant produced the most active principles. By preparing and extracting the oil from the hemp seeds, the researchers discovered for the first time a heretofore unknown source of the hallucinogen. Then, employing only the active principles, as opposed to the crude preparations commonly used by smokers, they injected the drug into animals to compare the results with the characteristic effects of the less refined form of marijuana.

It was known that the lethal dose for the unprepared cannabis drug was in the vicinity of two pounds of hashish. The researchers, however, claimed that such data had very little meaning. They found that 7,500 milligrams of the fluid extract were required to kill a frog; 1600 mgs, an albino mouse; and anywhere between 1700 to 5400 mgs, a dog. A significant discovery was made when they found that the pure preparation and the synthetics were not as toxic or dangerous as the crude preparations used by the public. They also found that the effects of these various preparations of cannabis in their crude form (such as marijuana, hashish, and *ganja*) were more complicated than the synthetics developed in the science laboratory.

While the synthetics showed some of the major effects of the more crude preparations, they did not produce all the effects. The scientists inferred, therefore, that a combination of various ingredients and substances, rather than one single chemical, accounted for the total effect of the cannabis. The specific isolated components only produced a certain part of the complete range of effects, such as the classic ataxia in the dog—a symptom later ascribed to the properties of tetrahydrocannabinol. They also found that a central stimulant such as the amphetamines—benzedrine and methedrine—considerably increased the ataxic action of marijuana.

Other findings relate to the stability of the drug. While early investigators concluded that the active principles of the drug were unstable (for this reason the sale of cannabis in some parts of India is limited by government control to preparations less than a year old), the La Guardia studies proved this to be false.

It was revealed that the hemp plant stacked in the open for several years had undiminished potency. They also found that distillate oils from the plant could be preserved for considerable periods of time. In an experiment with such oils, the scientists preserved one sample under seal at low temperature, while another was exposed to the air at room temperature. After two years, they found that the potency for the two batches was the same.

The latest study of the physiological and psychological effects of marijuana—actually, the first new controlled clinical research work done in the United States since the La Guardia Report—was carried out under the auspices of the Department of Psychiatry and Pharamacology at Boston University School of Medicine, which published its findings in the December 13, 1968 issue of *Science*. The object of the research team was to "define as clearly as possible in a neutral setting the pharmacological effects of the drug." It was headed by Andrew T. Weil, now an intern at the Mt. Zion Hospital in San Francisco, who spent several years studying the effects of marijuana and nutmeg, as well as Dr. Norman E. Zinberg, of Harvard, and Miss Judith M. Delson, of the Boston University School of Medicine.

The researchers tested two groups—nine "naive" subjects (men who had never turned on) and eight chronic marijuana users. Although their findings in the main are consistent with those of earlier investigations, the most striking information was the report of marijuana effects on the tyro volunteers, who apparently were hard to come by. Says the report: "It proved extremely difficult to find marijuana-naive persons in the student population of Boston . . . nearly all persons encountered who had not tried marijuana admitted this somewhat apologetically."

With the drug supplied by the Narcotics Bureau and rated for potency by a United States Customs laboratory, the researchers took all precautions to make the tests airtight. Dosage was carefully controlled, double-blind procedures were used (some subjects received placebos), while aerosol was sprayed in testing rooms to camouflage the smell of marijuana. The placebo joints contained leaves of the male hemp plant (which produces no high) to assure that the observations reported by the subjects would be due to marijuana and not to the subjects' expectations.

The naive subjects received three kinds of joints: one containing a high dose (two grams) of marijuana; one with a low dose (half a gram); and the placebo. Neither the subject nor the experimenter was told which cigarette was being smoked at which session. The regular users, however, were given only the high doses of marijuana in their tests.

The tests themselves were very similar to those used in the La Guardia study, consisting of a series of psychological and physiological measurements.

The findings for symptoms and behavior, organic and systemic functions, and psychophysical functions were very similar to those reported by the La Guardia investigators. The effects of one inhaled dose of marijuana reached maximum intensity within a half-hour, diminished after an hour, and disappeared within three hours. A moderate increase in heart rate (greater among regular users than among naive subjects) was also found, although the respiration rate and blood-sugar levels were not significantly affected. Somewhat surprisingly, no change in pupil size was recorded, but there was a reddening of the eyes, particularly among the regular users.

Naive subjects tested for psychophysical functions were found to suffer a small but significant impairment of their performance on simple tests. On the other hand, chronic marijuana smokers suffered no such impairment of performance. They had no difficulty matching symbols, responding to flashing letters, or keeping a stylus in contact with a small spot on a moving turntable. In fact, all of them did better on their tests as a result of smoking pot.

Dr. Weil explained this phenomenon as being due to the fact that regular smokers learn to "adapt to and overcome their performance deficits," and that "maintaining effective levels of performance for many tasks—driving, for example—is much easier under the influence of marijuana than under that of other psychoactive drugs (liquor, for instance)," since these drugs often give the user a false sense of improved functioning.

On the intellectual plane, the study revealed that after smoking marijuana the subjects had difficulty maintaining a logical line of thought. "They tended to go off on irrelevant tangents and forget what they started out to say," said Dr. Weil. He believes these results indicate that marijuana has a greater effect on the higher brain centers—those controlling thinking, perception, and mood—than on the lower brain centers, which control reflexes and coordination.

Regular and naive volunteers also differed in the spectrum of emotional reactions, the "heads" getting high more readily than the "straights," who appeared to have less intense subjective experiences. In other words, the regular users of marijuana got high on the same doses that had far less marked effects on the naive subjects. Only one of the nine men who had never before smoked pot got high after smoking a large dose. The report explained that naive subjects might have to undergo some sort of "pharmacological sensitization," i.e., they might require several experiences for the drug's effects to take hold.

The Boston University report concluded that "no adverse marijuana reactions occurred in any of our subjects," and that the drug is a "relatively mild intoxicant with minor, real, short-lived effects." Said Dr. Weil in a *New York Times* story about his research: "Medically, it's quite harmless. It's not like alcohol which can seriously injure, even kill, you. But I would not minimize the effects of marijuana on brain function."

As evidence that marijuana is nonaddictive, Weil pointed out that a follow-up study of the naive subjects six months after the experiment indicated that only two of the young men had subsequently tried marijuana on their own, and in each case only one time. Thus, he said, "We need not fear the moral implication of giving naive persons their first marijuana experience—a factor that is very important to future research on the subject."

Today pharmacology texts almost invariably classify cannabis as a hallucinogen—although a mild one—along with LSD, mescaline, psilocybin, and peyote. Researchers have found that marijuana, if taken in extremely potent doses, has effects similar to those of LSD, as the experiences reported by Baudelaire show. Almost all of the mind-altering phenomena associated with the more powerful hallucinogens can also be produced with inordinately high dosages of cannabis.

Dr. William McGlothlin, a Rand Corporation psychologist and drug expert, comments that "the wavelike aspect of the experience is almost invariably reported for cannabis as well as for all the other hallucinogens. Reports of perceiving various parts of the body as distorted, and depersonalization, or double consciousness, are very frequent, as well as spacial and temporal distortion. Visual hallucinations, seeing faces as grotesque, increased sensitivity to sound and merging of senses (synesthesia) are also common. Heightened suggestibility, perception of thinking more clearly and deeper awareness of the meaning of things are characteristic."

We again turn to *Marijuana: America's New Drug Problem,* by Dr. R. P. Walton: "The acute intoxication with hashish probably more nearly resembles that with mescaline than any of the other well-known drugs. Comparison with cocaine and the opiates does not bring out a very striking parallelism. With mescaline and hashish there are numerous common features which seem to differ only in degree."

Thus, the big difference between marijuana and the other hallucinogens would appear to be "only a matter of degree." By smoking marijuana the effects can be controlled and the desired state can be obtained at will. The French writer Michaux, who has experimented with various hallucinogens, writes that "compared to other hallucinogenic drugs, hashish is feeble, without great range, but easy to handle, convenient, repeatable without immediate danger." Marijuana, therefore, is popular with those not willing to hazard the unpredictable outcome of taking LSD, mescaline, or peyote; they can always count on pot as a "dependable producer of . . . euphoria and sense of well-being."

The mere action of puffing at a marijuana joint as noted by the La Guardia Report, is also considered by most users to be a more satisfying way of getting high than simply taking an oral dose. Oral ingestion, although not necessarily eliminating the feeling of euphoria, frequently gives rise to feelings of anxiety, irritability, and antagonism. As the report showed, smokers "learn" to use the drug effectively. Novices often have disappointing experiences with the drug, for by smoking too much they replace the pleasurable effects by feelings of paranoia and anxiety.

Since LSD and most other hallucinogens are not smoked, they are much less susceptible to directional restraint. Even a sophisticated user of the drug may find himself veering out of control and plunging into an agonizing welter of unpleasant sensations.

Another distinct difference between marijuana and the hallucinogens is the tendency for the former to act as a soporific drug and induce sleep. The other hallucinogens, on the contrary, tend to cause periods of wakefulness that last at least for the duration of their effects, which may vary from eight to twelve hours for LSD. At the same time, the two kinds of hallucinogens differ in their varying degrees of tolerance. Marijuana does not produce any tolerance at all; after the effects of the drug have worn off, an additional dose may be taken and the effects repeated. Regardless of the frequency and amount of marijuana smoked, no body of tolerance is built up.

This does not hold true for LSD or mescaline. These powerful drugs cannot usually induce their effects on the day following the "trip"; a waiting period from three to four days must commonly be observed before the full effects of the drug will again be apparent on ingestion of a dose. In addition, their hallucinogenic properties cannot be maintained for a period longer than that common to a single dose. The marijuana intoxication, however, can be sustained almost indefinitely by continuous smoking; in other words, the pothead can maintain a high for a day, two days, a week, or even a month, if he so desires, by smoking without cessation.

However, evidence from the use of these drugs supports the consensus that the marijuana smoker rarely indulges in such a prolonged exercise in the artificial stimulation of euphoria. Although he may indulge a number of times per week, he will not maintain a continuous high. Similarly, the overwhelming impact of the stronger hallucinogens, such as peyote and LSD, generally do not make the "tripper" want to repeat the experience at close intervals since the psychological hangover usually last much longer than the tolerant effect.

What does the aforementioned data gathered by various research groups mean to the casual marijuana smoker? The popular notion that the drug "heightens sensibility" is certainly borne out. The frequent dissolution of logical concepts under the influence of marijuana is often followed by a new look at the values imposed by society. The decrease in inhibition seems to be the result of this elimination of the social-value system, and the smoker seems to experience stimuli anew and with a much greater intensity. Thus calmness and the absence of unpleasant preoccupations and anxieties are essential to the marijuana experience and, in smoking with others, the company should be congenial. Irritations, too, are enhanced by the drug, which enormously increases all the sensibilities, both pleasant and unpleasant. The experiences under marijuana, as novelist William Burroughs points out, are very much dependent on the smoker's mood. Because marijuana intensifies one's original state of mind, "depression turns to despair, anxiety to panic, it makes a bad situation worse."

When the intake of the drug is controlled by the experienced smoker—like the social drinker who knows when he has had enough—the effects can usually be predicted and reactions such as anxiety are easily avoided. In this way the smoker restricts the effect to the euphoric state of consciousness, leaning back to observe his mind in action. The ideas that pass through the psyche seem at first to be uncontrollable, fantastic, and so rapid that for the novice smoker it is usually akin to a revelation. After awhile he will try to communicate these ideas, but since his mind works far more rapidly than his ability to verbalize, he may end up spouting fragments of sentences and incoherent verbiage. Whatever was on the mind of the individual before lighting up a joint is usually connected with the broken sequence of ideas going through his head. Concentration is impossible, though, and the mind tends to jump from one train of thought to another. It is very common for the smoker to stop in the middle of a sentence and ask his fellow smokers what he was talking about.

The evidence garnered by such reports as the La Guardia and

Boston University studies have done much to clear the cobwebs from the marijuana picture. A number of legal experts have advocated a legislation of control similar to that now reflected in the liquor regulations of the different states. The opposition to the drug's legalization continues to maintain that marijuana inevitably leads to the use of hard narcotics—heroin and/or cocaine.

There are other adverse problems involved in marijuana smoking, as already indicated by the findings elicited from the extensive testing employed in the La Guardia Report—symptoms experienced by many of the test individuals, and which included pressure in the head, difficulty in sustaining mental concentration, intellectual confusion, sluggish motor responses, occasional blurring of vision, cardiac palpitation, a reduction of drive, and frequent periods of anxiety.

Although it seems to be an accepted fact among most authorities that the drug does not alter the smoker's basic personality and is not addictive, there remains the very serious matter of its effect on the function of the brain. Perhaps, only time and additional medical research will reveal if there is danger of permanent brain damage from long and continued use of marijuana.

Why is marijuana, which may be so dangerous to the smoker, so popular? What is it in the experience that, once tasted, makes so many converts to its cause?

A contemporary marijuana smoker, a young man at Columbia University, explained in an interview with the authors what marijuana means to him. "Marijuana forces you to see what's happening. It turns you on by turning off the old restrictions that have been imposed upon you through years of living in the square world. All your thoughts, feelings, and sensations are new and strange. All events, physical, personal, or social are looked at with a new eye. You suddenly realize who you really are and what your personal reality means and when you see this you bring it back to the straight world and incorporate into your life whatever insights were gained by the experience.

"It is a psychedelic experience similar to LSD but on a lesser scale. It is consciousness expansion because it expands the scope of your personal reality. Until you have experienced the effects of the drug, you cannot know how narrow your previous ideas about the world were. The old stimuli seem to be magnified and come at you like gunshots and hit you with the same impact.

The old categorizing is forgotten and the walls and the masks that you have built up about you disappear. You suddenly get into closer contact with reality. You see many things; you see the phoniness, the superficiality, and the true personalities of others about you. You learn to appreciate the true value of things."

Such paeans to pot are not universally shared. Many educators and psychologists see the drug's use as a convenient cop-out from the responsibilities that accompany one's adjustment to society. Says Dr. Robert S. Liebert, psychiatric consultant at New York's Columbia University: ". . . when I talk to a kid who is turned on I have the sense of relating through a glass partition."

Few physicians, even those convinced of the safety of smoking marijuana, openly endorse its legalization for this very reason. "Our society," as Dr. Donald Louria, of New York's Cornell Medical College, says "has opted for enough escape mechanisms already—liquor, caffeine, and cigarettes." Like so many others of his colleagues, he sees marijuana as just another crutch to be added to the inventory of substances for evading reality.

CHAPTER FIVE

THE POT MYSTIQUE: HOW MARIJUANA IS USED

From Copping to the Tea-Pad Party

It is a rule of thumb that all animals shy away from pain and are drawn to that which gives them pleasure. Whether the indulgence is labeled a "crutch" or social "vice," if a growing segment of the population did not find it pleasurable, marijuana would not be as widespread as it is today. Today, there are few portions of the citizenry that do not count their smokers.

The situation as it exists at present bears little resemblance to the small groups of underprivileged marijuana smokers of fifty years ago. In the last few years it has spread rapidly among white middle-class youth and even among some of their elders. It is not, as is commonly supposed, used predominantly by the hippie element among youth, although it is a staple of their life's style. As a matter of fact, some hippies use LSD and amphetamines to a far greater extent than they do marijuana. It is the white middle-class college students who have been tagged "The Pot Generation." Marijuana is sometimes found almost as thick as the ivy on campuses throughout the nation and, according to recent stories in the popular press, it has now penetrated the high-school halls in our major cities as well.

At one time the virtual exclusive prerogative of the ghetto hipsters of the twenties, the remarkable thing about marijuana in the latter part of the sixties is that it has become mainly a middle-class phenomenon. Few today would be shocked to learn of a doctor with a busy practice in the city who occasionally relaxes by getting high with a group of friends. One of the more popular news magazines recently reported that more Americans than ever are turning on with marijuana. Most of them are under twenty-one, but an astonishing number are respectable adult citizens.

It is difficult to determine the total, but James L. Goddard, former commissioner of the United States Food and Drug Administration, estimates that as many as twenty million Americans may have used marijuana at one time or another, while four hundred thousand—some say as many as three million—may now be smoking it regularly. Other estimates put the total of occasional users from three to five million, with regular users ranging between a half-million to one million. Its illegality, coupled with its new widespread use among all strata of society, has produced what must be called a marijuana subculture.

Those who share the experiences and problems of procurement and safety are held together by a bond that crosses racial, class, and age lines. At the same time, as its use filters into more and more different levels of the population, the smoker who emerges comes closer to a representative American type. The young, the minorities, the alienated, the fringe-group members, and the liberals are, nevertheless, still over-represented. In *Marijuana: Myths and Realities,* J. L. Simmons, a sociologist at the University of California, estimates that every passing week fifty thousand new people per week try marijuana in this country—perhaps the fastest-growing group to join the quarter of a billion cannabis users throughout the world.

The current spate of news reports, magazine articles, television programs, and sociological studies dealing with the herb and its growing legion of devotees reflects marijuana's increasing popularity. Pot, so the glossy weeklies tell us, has become an American fact of life.

A subterranean culture, with its own underground newpsapers, films, radio and TV stations, is closely tied to the phenomenon of illicit drug use in the United States. The Beatles have found an older audience, not only through the evolution of their music, but to a lesser degree for their public advocacy of legalized pot in England.

Because pot heightens the senses—including hearing—smokers buy not only classical and jazz records, but have helped to make popular the psychedelic rock of dozens of new groups—the

Doors, the Mothers of Invention, Country Joe and the Fish, and the Jefferson Airplane. There can be no question but that these sudden new developments in musical tastes and other art forms have been influenced, at least to some extent, by an increasing use of marijuana over the past five years by persons in all walks of life. In this period, the drug subculture has spawned an intellectual and religious mystique entirely unlike the abuse exemplified by the spread of heroin addiction during the 1930's.

Police no longer find themselves facing the hopeless addict and alienated junkie whose "habit" determines a predictable behavior pattern; more and more frequently they are encountering an enlightened person whose use of drugs is a result of free choice. Although the authorities continue to identify the drug user with all anti-Establishment forces because that choice is contrary to popular mores, the smoker today comes from all classes of society and one particular group can no longer be tagged as the chief user and purveyor of marijuana. There is no "type" of person who smokes marijuana any more than there is a "type" of person who takes a drink. Nowadays anyone can be a smoker —from the college student and college graduate who picked up the habit in college, through the whole spectrum of American life—scientists, mailmen, factory workers, and just about any other "type."

If there are still misconceptions surrounding marijuana they reside primarily in the over-forty group, which never had the chance to come into contact with the drug in their youth and were brought up on the myth propagated in the thirties and forties. Although they have a very small percentage of smokers among them, the latest evidence shows that the practice is growing as the younger generation exposes and introduces them to the drug. Records of arrest are a misleading indication of the type of person who turns on since the young often tend to be indiscreet in their smoking and copping habits.

Since there are stringent legal obstacles to the use, sale, and procurement of marijuana, its distribution is limited to sources not readily available to the ordinary person. The pot smoker is the final link in a chain of supply usually made up of individuals and groups operating outside the bounds of conventional society. Contacts, however, leading to possible supply sources, known as "connections," are usually not hard to make. These initial maneuverings leading to the first smoke provide the basis for a level of occasional use in which the individual smokes pot sporadically and irregularly. Then, unless he is with others who have a supply, he may cease smoking it and remain on the fringe of the marijuana crowd. He may or may not have liked the experience, but most likely he'll feel obliged not to turn down an offer to indulge. He is unlikely to keep a supply of marijuana himself, and when he does share a joint, his decision is dictated by social reasons, just as the nondrinker does not mind taking a "shot" at a cocktail party or night club.

Not averse to those who do smoke, the casual smoker will certainly never express his disapproval or become alarmed by those who make it a regular practice. However, if he has more than a passing liking for the experience, he may purchase a supply if the opportunity presents itself and usually smoke it within a few days in the company of friends who are similarly inclined.

It is clear, then, that as a social relaxer marijuana is favored for the same reasons as is alcohol by an older generation, despite the fact that the former is much more difficult to obtain. The smoker of marijuana usually finds his friends among like-minded persons whose attitude towards the drug corresponds to his own. It goes without saying that one could never feel at ease when smoking in the company of someone violently opposed to its use. In the parlance of pot, this would be a "bring-down."

The occasional smoker who becomes more regular in his practice will eventually turn to those of a similar bent of mind since they represent the stable source of supply he needs. Although it may not be his original intention, once the casual smoker has laid in a supply he is on his way to becoming a regular smoker. If he is continually turned on by his crowd, he'll feel obliged to reciprocate and subsequently keep a supply handy for the occasion.

A more frequent smoker may light up as often as once or twice a week, usually with members of his immediate circle of friends. With the appearance in large numbers of the middle-class smoker, the person who turns on occasionally today probably constitutes the bulk of marijuana users in this country. More likely than not, he is a sensible individual who pays careful attention to the legal restrictions and will go out of his way to avoid being detected. He won't consider his practice a vice, but he is aware of the stigma society at large still attaches to the habit and his use is likely to be moderate for those reasons. His position is very similar to that of the person who kept a supply of alcoholic beverages during the Prohibition era. But unlike the drinker, who does not suffer from social disapproval, the occasional smoker leads a double life—his normal, everyday life with occupations and interests that far outrank his interest in marijuana (unlike the pothead, who will be discussed later), and his secret life involving his smoking activities. This citizen usually justifies his indulgence by claiming that the law is unrealistic and that he therefore sees no reason to be bound by it.

From the above, we may infer that there are three types of marijuana smokers—the casual smoker, the social smoker, and the pothead.

The casual and the social smoker are distinguished by a difference of degree—the difference between the individual who occasionally lays in a couple of bottles of beer and the person whose social life is built around drinking. Although he may go without it for a considerable length of time, the social smoker prefers to keep some marijuana around the house. He is usually a secure person who does not feel he has to prove anything by turning on, as is often the case with the younger generation. More often than not, he is considered successful in conventional terms. Having picked up the habit in the military or in college, he continues it with the knowledge that there are far more important things in his life.

If his wife knows of this practice she may raise objections, although they are apt to be disregarded. In such a situation, the husband who prefers domestic peace above all usually keeps his supply hidden, rolling a joint when she is absent. It is unusual, but not uncommon, that if the facilities are available he may grow a little patch of his own and harvest its yield several times a year. This practice, though, is more likely among the potheads. Because the social smoker has to think of his family and career, he takes pains to be extremely discreet and is sure to take the maximum precautions before smoking.

The most inveterate smoker is the pothead. Smoking daily and sometimes staying high for days on end, he builds his whole life around getting stoned on marijuana. Although his habit is not a physical dependence like that of the heroin addict or the alcoholic, he is similar to the problem drinker who does not want to stop "lushing it up." To the pothead any contact with reality is a bring-down and for this reason he is happiest when he is high.

There are, in addition, other kinds of heads—"hashheads," who smoke hashish out of tiny pipes with long stems, aiming beyond the "buzz" and the high to the timeless "zonk." The cognoscenti among them may avail themselves of a *chillum*—a cylindrical pipe used in India with a small bowl on top of the stem. The hash is smoked by holding the pipe vertically and drawing at its narrow bottom, which is wrapped in a thin piece of moist cloth.

The pothead gets stoned by smoking an average of at least an hour each day, puffing away at anywhere from one to ten cigarettes. He maintains a supply of marijuana at home and turns on whenever he feels like it. His life revolves almost completely around his habit. His friends smoke and he shares their attitudes, their habits, their smoking techniques, and their outlook on the square world, which is pitied for its ignorance of the pleasures of being high all the time. He is likely to feel disdain for those who condemn his practice or find greater satisfaction in carrying on their daily tasks. The pothead considers them "up-tight"—anxiety-ridden. One of his beliefs is that more of today's eminent men and show-business personalities turn on than the public knows about.

Virtually all of his time is taken up by smoking or thinking about it and copping new and/or better supplies. His habit directs his life to the exclusion of everything that interferes with it. If his work or school studies do not present a threat to getting stoned when the fancy strikes him, he is likely to continue them. If they do interfere, they must go. From then on, he'll try to survive by his wits, taking odd jobs or becoming a pusher himself. He thinks of himself as a dropout from society, although he considers junkies addicted to hard narcotics as "dumb" and "silly" for getting trapped into a situation they can't control. He doesn't think of his marijuana habit as an addiction. He sees it as his way of showing his emancipation from the dictates of society and a means of defining his attitude toward reality.

The pothead is a relative newcomer on the drug scene. Like his more seriously addicted predecessor—the junkie—he is alienated from society, but never to the extent that he can't bridge the gap to the straight world. He is usually a person in his late teens or early twenties who is trying to come to grips with himself and society. His hang-ups are those usually associated with the young in their attempt to appraise the values and concepts they grew up with.

Once he has settled these conflicts, he usually does not remain a pothead much longer. He will gradually diminish his smoking as he finds new interests and his place in society. After a year or two at the most, he will have cut down to the level of the social smoker. He will have discovered that the pleasures of marijuana are greatest when enjoyed in moderation, making each turn-on a fresh departure from the everyday instead of the unvaried soporific confusion of his days as a pothead. But aside from these reasons, he will have probably tired of his underground existence with its constant worries over police "busts."

If he embarks on a career, he may find it increasingly difficult to keep up the double life in and outside the social boundaries. He may have come to realize that nonconformity can be expressed in any number of ways besides that of the cop-out of the confirmed pothead. Although it is unlikely that he will cease smoking altogether, he will relegate the activity to its proper place in his life.

When the pothead cops his purchase of marijuana, he prefers to buy in large amounts from a seller he can deal with directly. In this way he eliminates the added cost of the middleman. At the same time, by purchasing a large quantity he obtains the goods at a reduced price.

However, before he can cop he has to know a connection. Pushers, with good reason, are more paranoid about the police than anything else and they'll refuse to do business unless the buyer is identified to them in a way that arouses no suspicion. For the person remote from the drug scene, finding the connection is not easy. Involvement and identification with a group of smokers is usually the only way to solve his problem. Acceptance by such a group indicates that he can be trusted to buy drugs without jeopardizing anyone else. The novice, however, usually hesitates to do so at first for fear of arrest. Dealers are notorious for attracting the police, who are known to wait until they have the goods on as many persons as possible. But once a purchase has been made without any trouble, such fears are commonly no longer operative and the activity becomes routine with its own geography of meeting places and mystique of caution.

The ease or difficulty experienced in copping depends on

whether the buyer is a casual smoker, social smoker, or a pothead. Each of these categories has its corresponding mystique. Once a person learns the drug geography in his town or city, he usually knows the pusher and can always contact him with a minimum of fuss.

It is more difficult for the casual smoker unfamiliar with the pot terrain. The approach and language used by a prospective buyer in contacting a connection for the first time serves to give the dealer a fair impression on which to proceed. The connection often knows intuitively whether the buyer's pitch is genuine or the cover of a police agent.

It has been shown that the pothead lives in a subculture with its own life style, language, rituals, and paranoias. It's especially the latter, whether real or imagined, that imparts to his life its pervasive character—often the result of deliberate cultivation for without it much of the head's raison d'être would be meaningless.

As noted previously, his indulgence in marijuana is in many ways a stance of defiance against the Establishment forces. Were it not for his belief that society, as embodied by the law enforcers, is constantly out to get him, he might well seek some other way of expressing his rebellion. Anyone who has ever been around heads knows that the frequent stupid risks they take give the appearance that they are actually inviting arrest. Psychologists have noted that a certain element of lawbreakers share a self-destructive tendency that is only satisfied by being apprehended. Since only a modicum of circumspection is required to avoid detection in smoking marijuana, the pothead who is "busted" usually falls into this category.

Prior to smoking, doors are carefully locked, curtains are drawn tight, while some even go so far as to paint the windows black to foil the police from noticing the red lights favored by potheads. Today's cult of "stashing" the marijuana hails from the days of comparatively fewer smokers when the consequently greater chance of being caught led the head to look for ingenious hiding places for his supply of marijuana.

They would "stash" the pot by concealing it in such places as the toilet tank, under loose floor boards or tiles, behind the plate of a light switch, or in a variety of holes as artfully crafted as a set of Chinese boxes. Before stashing it, some would even take the precaution of wrapping the drug in a substance such as lard, which neutralizes the smell of pot and helps to throw the police off scent. Others prefer to hide their contraband outside the home—in the hollow of a tree, on the rooftop, on a stairway landing, in the backyard, or in a locker at a bus or air terminal.

Rolling a marijuana cigarette is similar to the technique for rolling an ordinary cigarette, although the joint, "stick," or "reefer" is with a few exceptions considerably thinner—about half the diameter of an ordinary tobacco cigarette. Some dexterity is needed to prevent the loose marijuana tobacco from spilling. For this reason the ends of the cigarette papers used are usually twisted together to pack the "grass" into a relatively solid cigarette.

The La Guardia Report described how an earlier generation of pot smokers rolled their cigarettes. In the main it was similar to the manner used today—two gum-edged cigarette papers stuck together with saliva from the tongue and then rolled with the ends twisted together. The old practice was to wet the whole cigarette with saliva for the purpose of making the joint burn slowly. This is not done today simply for hygienic reasons and possibly because the present generation of smokers is more affluent than its forerunner. The thin cigarette, though, is still in vogue since it allows maximum consumption of the marijuana whereas much of the smoke of a regular-size joint goes to waste. The two papers also continue to be used, not only because they make the cigarette easier to roll but because they make it burn more slowly as well. Recently some smokers have begun using cigarette-making machines that produce a joint that looks exactly like a regular cigarette.

The La Guardia Report mentions that at the time the study was made, there were instances where the marijuana tobacco was chewed with the same effect as might be obtained through smoking. Of course, in those days chewing ordinary tobacco was far more popular than it is today and the potheads who favored this practice were merely continuing a custom of their time.

Potheads claim that marijuana, like wine, comes in different varieties—some superb, some good, some terrible. But because only a few kinds are readily accessible, most pot smokers have only sampled the more common types of grass that find their way into this country across the Mexican-American border. The staple for American smokers is green Mexican grass of reputedly ordinary quality. Of a lesser quality is the polluted variety grown in window boxes and on rooftops by more economy-minded city dwellers.

If there are numerous kinds of grass, there are just as many kinds of papers to roll it in. The most famous are the white Zig-Zag papers whose covers feature the well-known bearded face, the manufacturer's trademark that recently has been reproduced on pop posters, tee-shirts, and buttons as a campy put-on of the square world, a symbol recognized by potheads all over the country. The face with the beard turns up on posters with marijuana leaves above and below his face; the Mouse Studios of San Francisco (a hippie art studio) sell "Zig-Zag Man" tee-shirts, available in such colors as Acapulco gold, Panama red, and Guadalajara green.

Potheads however, use dozens of roll-your-own cigarette papers, including Marfil and Bambu, both from Spain, Rizzla-Plus from France, Papel de Arroz from Mexico, licorice-flavored Stella from England, and Top, manufactured in the United States. (Hippies are eager to point out that "Top" is "pot" spelled backward).

Depending on the size of his pocketbook, the smoker today may roll what is called a "bomb" (about the size of a regular cigarette), or a "cigar" (a marijuana cigarette close to the size of a cigar). On the West Coast, with its more plentiful availability of marijuana, joints are rolled much fatter than they are in New York where smokers prefer the skinny joints for economical reasons.

Smokers on the more affluent West Coast are also in the habit of tossing away "roaches" (the butts of marijuana cigarettes) contrary to the practice on the East Coast where they are scrupulously saved for a rainy day. The true pothead, however, values roaches for another reason: He believes that the potency gathers in a roach so that it is the last third of a marijuana cigarette that packs the biggest punch.

As continuous puffing reduces the marijuana cigarette until it can no longer be held comfortably with the fingers, it ceases being a joint and becomes a roach; the tars and resins, having filtered towards the rear of the cigarette, cause the butt to turn brownish, resembling a cockroach in size, shape, and color. Depending on the size, length, and potency of the joint as well as its thickness, the strength of the roach can be as much as half a full-size marijuana cigarette. Heads are naturally loathe to see such a delight go to waste, and a number of ingenious instruments called "roach holders" have been perfected by the pot underground in answer to the problem.

The "cocktail" method—one of the most popular means of consuming roaches—involves the removal of about an inch of tobacco from a regular cigarette. The roach is then inserted in the emptied part and the paper twisted around it. Its chief disadvantage is that the regular cigarette tobacco filters the marijuana smoke, reducing his potency and subsequent effects.

The "opium pipe," which can be purchased in the Chinatown of almost any city, adds a little more class to the roach holder. Usually sold as a souvenir or cigarette holder, it consists of a brass bowl that is about a half-inch in diameter and fastened to a long bamboo stem. The roach is easily fitted into the bowl and as the marijuana is drawn it further benefits from the foot-long stem, which helps to cool the smoke to a less searing quality.

Some of the other methods practiced are adaptations from the various ways of holding ordinary cigarette butts developed by hobos, such as sticking a pin through the butt to avoid burning the fingers. The pothead utilizes anything that will do the same for holding the roach. He uses paper clips, nails, tie clips, hair clips, stickpins, bobby pins, tweezers, pliers, forceps, and even the clip of a ballpoint pen.

Many marijuana users favor pipes, claiming that it's not only a better way to smoke but also prevents unnecessary waste of pot. There are literally hundreds of varieties of pipes employed for this purpose—short ones, long ones, pipes made of plumbing fixtures, clay, wood, brass, ebony, and stone. A typical stone pipe resembles an inverted pyramid with two holes, one for inhaling, the other to hold the marijuana; it can be comfortably held with two hands and the larger opening is easily covered to prevent loss of smoke when passing the pipe, or between inhalations. More exotic—and said to be more satisfying—are the water pipes, such as hookahs, or narghiles. These are reputed to let the smoke travel farther and thus make it milder by passing it through water in the base of the pipe.

Some people who do not smoke, or women who find the searing smoke of the marijuana cigarette unpleasant, have formulated recipes to make it more palatable as an ingredient in ordinary foodstuffs. Gertrude Stein, patroness of the expatriate American literary establishment in Paris of the twenties, knew that marijuana can be mixed with such foods as salads and brownies. Her lifelong companion, Alice B. Toklas, included a recipe for hashish fudge in her cookbook. She said that anyone could whip it up on a rainy day and recommended it as an "entertaining refreshment for a ladies' bridge club or a chapter meeting of the Daughters of the American Republic."

Among other preparations known in the United States is marijuana tea. Sugar is added and the tea is drunk hot. Marijuana is also baked in the form of cake and cookies by being first crushed to a fine powder, which is then added to ordinary cake mix or kneaded into a batch of cookie dough.

Hippies have not been long in adopting the various preparations popular in India. The marijuana tea known in that country as *bhang* is becoming popular among hippies who brew it on festive occasions, such as weddings. Mint is sometimes added to enhance the flavor. Indians usually add the marijuana to food in the form of a liquid or paste, which is made by boiling marijuana leaves until there is no water left.

In the Middle East this same paste may be added to various types of drinks, sometimes to alcoholic beverages such as wine. As a spawning ground for delicacies containing marijuana paste, the Middle East is unsurpassed with such prized concoctions as peanut brittle (*manzul*), honey-and-nut cookies (*majun*), and another type of peanut-butter candy (*garawash*). The paste is also stuffed in dates and added to Turkish Delight.

American students who have traveled in North Africa have become the innovators on the United States drug scene by bringing marijuana out of the joint or pipe and into the kitchen. The effects of marijuana eaten as "brownies" or otherwise are much longer in coming, usually about an hour after ingestion. With smoking the effects usually begin manifesting themselves in about five or ten minutes.

The La Guardia Report field investigators did not offer such tasty morsels as are preferred by today's more culinary-inclined potheads. They did, however, submit copious comments on the habits of marijuana smoking, which in the intervening twenty-five years have not undergone any remarkable changes. A glance at the report's sociological findings shows that the smoking ritual has been adopted virtually intact by today's potheads. Like the early tea-pad patrons, the novice smoker learns by observing others. Thus he masters the method of inhaling the marijuana cigarette.

They also noted a custom known as "pick-up" smoking—a practice similar to the one popular today in which the joint is passed around after being lit by a smoker who takes one or two inhalations and then gives it to the next person. This procedure, they observed, was repeated until all present had had an opportunity to take a puff or two of the cigarette. They also recorded that the confirmed marijuana smoker consumed perhaps from six to ten cigarettes per day and appeared to be quite conscious of the quantity he required to reach the effect called high. The smoker recognized this point as an onset of various forms of anxiety that he would immediately quash by taking a number of measures enabling him to "come down." This explained the need for such beverages as beer or sweet soda pop.

The smokers interviewed emphasized that the consumption of whiskey neutralizes the potency of the drug and that for this reason smokers would not drink while "blowing" marijuana. On the other hand, sweet wine does not seem to be incompatible with pot and experienced smokers agree that this mild alcoholic beverage aids the drug in producing the desired effects.

The main difference between the generations of potheads is in the "setting" as shown in the disappearance today of the tea pad in which the pusher of a quarter-century ago supplied not only the drug itself but also a place with an atmosphere similar to a neighborhood tavern. The independent pot peddlers were around then as well and together with the tea pad they constituted the two main channels for the distribution of marijuana.

At the time of the report in 1944, there were about five hundred such tea pads in Harlem and at least five hundred peddlers. The tea pad consisted of a room or an apartment in which the people gathered to smoke marijuana. It was furnished according to the clientele it expected to serve. The lighting was more or less uniformly dim with blue predominating, incense was considered part of the furnishing, and the walls were frequently decorated with pictures of nude subjects.

The report states that the marijuana smoker seemed to derive greater satisfaction from smoking in the presence of others, and the atmosphere of the tea pad was precisely to create that atmosphere of comfort and restful ease. The attitude of a smoker in a tea pad was that of a relaxed individual, free from the anxieties and cares of life.

The researchers also discovered an interesting arrangement that was clearly not along orthodox lines from a business standpoint. This was a series of pup tents, each series pitched on a rooftop of an apartment building in Harlem. The smokers turned on in the tents, and upon feeling sufficiently high they emerged into the open to discuss and admire the stars and the wonders of the universe.

The La Guardia Report also found that marijuana smoking was very common in the theatres of Harlem. In some instances, employees of the theatres actually sold marijuana cigarettes on the premises. In the Harlem dance halls, the patrons as well as the musicians were frequently observed to be lighting up in the lavatories or around the main floor. There was no evidence that the sales being made by the employees on the premises were profitable to the owners of the theatres—or that they were even aware of this practice. Nothing, however, was done to prohibit it. Other methods of retail distribution centered around a few select places, usually bars and grills, restaurants, and neighborhood stores. It could also be bought from terminal porters.

The La Guardia researchers further learned about the preferred setting for smoking marijuana from the volunteers tested. They were quoted as saying that they enjoyed the drug more in a less clinical atmosphere than that provided by the hospital. Therefore, in order to observe the drug's effects in a more natural environment and in less formal circumstances, several get-togethers were arranged to approximate the style of the tea pad. The smokers were consulted beforehand and the stage was set according to the volunteers' wishes. They requested easy chairs or floor cushions and that the party not begin until it was totally dark outside. Then the radio was turned to soft dance music as one shaded light bulb burned and the greater part of the room became washed with shadows.

Today the setting has not changed much. When Dr. Leary and a group of his friends were arrested in upstate New York for possession of hallucinogens a few years ago, the setting was almost identical to that suggested by the smokers in the La Guardia Report. There were pillows scattered about the floor and the music consisted of Indian *ragas*. Dim lights, music, a generally congenial atmosphere seem to be among the main ingredients that go into the successful setting of the pot party as well as the LSD trip.

Although it has been noted in the beginning of this chapter that the use of marijuana today has become a middle-class phenomenon with its rapid spread to the over-twenty-five generation, it is the young who have been mainly responsible for its growing acceptance by all segments of the population. They look on pot as a liberator of feelings and perceptions, which they see increasingly stifled and channeled into molds shaped by the inexorable pressures of a complex, technologically oriented society.

Despite the seeming freedom given to modern man by our sophisticated communication media and supersonic travel, the young feel that the individual pays for these questionable benefits by being stamped into a tintype of standard uniformity. They see pot as blowing smoke into the eyes of the forces that mold conformity. Many bright young men and women have turned away from what they call the rat race—a type of existence that they regard as essentially meaningless and a betrayal of the perception of life as an unfolding experience of emotional and esthetic growth.

Every generation of young Americans has had its groups of restless and idealistic individuals who have always found a way of sublimating these feelings—through a country pushing westward, making the world safe for democracy, the New Deal, Kennedy's New Frontier. Today, the young see no such avenues open to them. Although not necessarily abandoning the causes, studies, or work they find worthwhile, they are increasingly turned inward, "getting into their own heads." Apart from this factor, many of those who turn on belong to the bored and frustrated. Unprecedented affluence has deprived them of the need to scramble for their economic place in society. At the same time they feel powerless to influence the events of the day—the war in Vietnam, slums and poverty in the cities, the draft, and the futility of protest opposed at every turn by the massive forces of constituted authority. To many, the relief of dropping out—if only temporarily—is a tempting one. Marijuana makes such an action seem easy.

A great many of the casual smokers are involved in creative or artistic endeavors. The question whether or not marijuana tends to influence creativity is a moot point. The fact remains, however, that a great many artists as well as members of other fringe groups include a disproportionate number of marijuana smokers. They share many of the hang-ups common to the young and, like them, they are skeptical of the values espoused by straight society. They are also more susceptible to the anguish of the times and more sensitive to the problems facing them.

Marijuana offers a temporary release from the bondage of these frustrations and it is exactly this effect of pot that has provided the main stock of ammunition to those opposing its use—the claim that it keeps the person suspended in a state of limbo and prevents him from seeking his proper station in life. Proponents of the drug insist, however, that such fears are groundless. Relatively few of those smoking casually or socially become confirmed heads; and Dr. David H. Powelson, Chief of Psychiatric Services at the University of California at Berkeley, observes that, "the question of what would happen to society if everyone used pot assumes that if some people use it, everyone will use it. It has always been generally available and still only a few use it."

Sociologists concur that marijuana is part of a continuing revolutionary cycle among the young to experiment with the new and be contemptuous of the old. The young themselves, whether they smoke or not, feel themselves above the controversy.

Had marijuana been legalized thirty years ago when it first became an issue, much of the steam of the present conflict would have evaporated a long time ago. It is particularly curious, the young generation points out, that a society that does not turn away from cigarettes and alcohol frowns upon marijuana. Adapting H. L. Mencken's observation about pornography that no girl has ever been ruined by a dirty book, marijuana users say that its legalization would pose no threat to society at large or individuals in particular.

Most of those who argue for keeping those laws in force base their reasoning on the contention that more research is needed before we can tell how dangerous over the long term marijuana smoking is. Ferdinand Mount, in an article titled, "The Wild Grass Chase," in *National Review* of January, 1968, opposes legalization on the grounds that a minority of the psychically weak and emotionally unstable need to be protected from the psychotic state and anxiety that occasionally attend marijuana smoking. He remarks that in a case where medical opinion is as divided as it is on the pros and cons of pot, "it would be crazy to act other than with extreme caution."

He refutes the argument that the drug's legalization would not alarmingly increase the number of users by drawing a logical connection between its accessibility and consequent indulgence. Present laws, he writes, serve as a deterrent to many young people who, under less restrictive circumstances, might easily become habitual users. Says Mount: "The argument that marijuana is no worse in its effects than alcohol . . . hardly justifies the legalization of marijuana on health grounds. And it would only justify legalization on the ground that laws must operate with the consent of the governed if the marijuana laws approached the unpopularity of Prohibition."

CHAPTER SIX

IS POT SAFE? THE MEDICAL PICTURE

The Dangers, the Question of Addiction, the Heroin Problem

Is marijuana dangerous? . . . Does indulgence beat an inevitable path to the insane asylum? . . . Does it make psychotics out of previously normal persons? . . . Does it do permanent damage to the mind? . . . Is it habit-forming—that is, does it build up an overriding need for continued use? . . . And does its use inevitably lead to heroin addiction? In short, do all the stories that have been current in the United States for more than fifty years add up to a grand old wives' tale or are they to be taken at face value?

The truth, as always, lies somewhere in between.

Whether or not marijuana is harmful to the user has been the subject of intensive medical research both in this country and abroad. Its legend of crime, insanity, and addiction has made it a veritable specter, stalked by the mass media and earnest medical forums in a continuous debate over the drug's pros and cons.

At the same time, although the evidence is not yet complete, there seems to be general accord that the drug does not fall into the narcotics category and does not inevitably lead to addiction or physical dependence on the hard narcotics. Instead, many medical authorities are becoming increasingly convinced that cannabis is no more dangerous than tobacco and no more habit-forming than liquor. In fact, much of the opinion holds that it is less dangerous and less habit-forming than our two most popular "vices." This view has been backed up by former United

States Food and Drug Administration Commissioner James L. Goddard.

"Whether or not marijuana is a more dangerous drug than alcohol is debatable," he said as commissioner. "I don't happen to think it is."

Dr. James M. Fox, while Director of the Bureau of Drug Abuse, indicated a similar view in a 1966 statement: "I think we can now say that marijuana does not lead to degeneration, does not affect the brain cells, is not habit-forming and does not lead to heroin addiction."

Borrowing a leaf from these and similar views, the President's Commission on Law Enforcement and the Administration of Justice, plumped for the liberal marijuana view in a statement issued in 1967: "Marijuana is equated in the law with the opiates, but the abuse characteristics of the two have almost nothing in common. The opiates produce physical dependence. Marijuana does not. A withdrawal sickness appears when the use of opiates is discontinued. No such symptoms are associated with marijuana. The desired dose of opiates tends to increase over time, where this is not true of marijuana."

Similar statements have been made by a number of other competent investigators. Going against the stream of such authoritative opinion, law-enforcement officials—especially those of the Bureau of Narcotics—and the mass media still cling to sharply divergent views.

The opinions of the anti-marijuana forces are well-exemplified by the statements that have been made periodically by officials directly, or indirectly, connected with perpetuating the drug's taboo status in the American pharmacopoeia. The Federal Bureau of Narcotics Commissioner declared in 1953 that marijuana "has no therapeutic value and its use is therefore always an abuse and a vice. This important fact should never be forgotten." Psychologist Martin Hoffman, writing in the *Yale Review* in 1964, pointed out the illogic behind such reasoning. "Many things," he wrote, "have no current therapeutic value—cabbage for one—although their use is therefore not to be considered a vice, and calling something an 'abuse and a vice' is not an 'important fact'; it is not a fact at all, but a moral judgment."

For one thing, as early as 1937, the drug was being considered for a variety of therapeutic uses. Dr. Robert Walton, in

Marijuana: America's New Drug Problem, made a sober assessment of its medical possibilities regarding therapeutic application:

> Although the hemp preparations may have been used by the ancients to produce anesthesia, these drugs were not generally introduced into medicine until about 1840. At this time, O'Shaughnessy, Aubert Roche, and Moreau de Tours observed its use in India and Egypt and proceeded to experiment with its therapeutic possibilities. After using it in different sorts of conditions, they were each enthusiastic in representing it as a valuable therapeutic agent. Their activities resulted in a very widespread and general use of the drug in both Europe and America. During the period 1840-1900 there were something over one hundred articles published which recommended cannabis for one disorder or another.

Walton agrees that the unsavory reputation the drug developed did much to diminish its medicinal potential:

> Cannabis preparations have come to occupy so minor a place among modern medicinals that it has been suggested that they be abandoned altogether, this latter point of view being based on the assumption that they represent a menace from the standpoint of the hashish habit. Such an action would certainly be too drastic in view of the circumstances. For one thing, the therapeutic use of cannabis and the hashish habit are almost entirely unrelated.

Some of the therapeutic uses he mentions were in the treatment of cough, fatigue, rheumatism, rheumatic neuralgia, asthma, and delirium tremens. Walton quotes several other doctors who claim that the drug gives relief from pain and migraine, and mentions several other medicinal uses for marijuana—in uterine dysfunction, painful and excessive menstruation, impaired labor and childbirth. Regarding the last two uses of the drug, he refers to a paper published in the *Journal of the American Medical Association* that credits cannabis with analgesic properties making childbirth less painful for the woman in labor by reducing the acuteness of touch and inducing a tranquil sleep. "As far as is known," he writes, "a baby born of a mother intoxicated with cannabis will not be abnormal in any way." He further noted the use of cannabis in psychological therapy by examining the reports of a number of doctors who had employed it for this purpose. In cases of depressive mental conditions, he found most of the cannabis experimenters in agreement that the drug benefited the patients treated.

Dr. Victor Robinson, a physician and chemist who is also one of the leading experts on cannabis, corroborated the therapeutic history of marijuana explored by Walton. In an essay in *Ciba Symposia* entitled "Concerning Cannabis Indica," Robinson traces the many medicinal uses to which the drug has been put:

> In the most ancient of all medical works, the *Susruta Samhita,* hemp is recommended for catarrh. A Sanskrit work on materia medica, *Rajbulubha,* alludes to the use of hemp in gonorrhea. In the first century, Dioscorides—the most renowned of the ancient writers on materia medica—recommended the seeds in the form of a cataplasm to soothe inflammation. Galen wrote that it is customary to give hemp to guests at banquets to promote hilarity and happiness. At the beginning of the third century, the Chinese physician Hoa-Thoa used hemp as an anesthetic in surgical operations.

Among other medicinal applications of cannabis, Dr. Robinson lists its use in the cure of alcoholics and morphine addicts, hysteria, nervous vomiting, St. Vitus' dance, epileptic fits, locomotor ataxia, hydrophobia, softening of the brain, and hemorrhage occurring in the final cessation of the menses.

Despite the many attempts to ban the drug in countries around the world, it continues to be used today as a popular euphoriant and medicinal agent. Its therapeutic uses have been developed especially in such countries and areas as the West Indies, Africa, Latin America, East Asia, and India as part of the folk medicine practiced in hundreds of villages lacking ready access to modern hospital care.

During the last hundred years more has been learned in the Western countries about its medicinal aspects. Prior to its ban, it was prescribed for sedation, senile insomnia, menstrual disorders, epilepsy, severe neuralgia, and migraine. Dr. Tod M. Mikuriya, a psychiatrist in private practice in San Francisco, who also served as a consultant on cannabis research to the National Institute of Mental Health, has given close scrutiny to the drug's history here.

All the evidence from a century of medicinal use, according to Dr. Mikuriya, clearly shows that the drug is not a narcotic in the medical sense. Since it is not physiologically addicting, says Dr. Mikuriya, there are no withdrawal pains. There is little or no build-up or tolerance that would lead to the use of increasing doses, as is the case with the true narcotics (opium and its refined extracts, heroin, morphine, codeine) and their synthetic substitutes. In addition, Dr. Mikuriya reported cannabis to be so nearly nontoxic that to kill one mouse requires forty thousand times the dose necessary to produce the state known as high in a human. By contrast, only twenty times the relaxant dose of alcohol can kill a man.

The La Guardia Report, by the very nature of its thoroughgoing research and independently drawn conclusions, served to dispel some of the nation's fears about marijuana, although it did point out some adverse and unfavorable symptoms as they occurred in tested individuals. Opponents of the drug, however, remained largely unconvinced that it could safely be indulged by the public at large. On April 28, 1945, for example, the *Journal of the American Medical Association* editorally assailed the report:

> The book states unqualifiedly to the public that the use of this narcotic does not lead to physical, mental, or moral degeneration and that permanent deleterious effects from its continued use were not observed on seventy-seven prisoners. This statement has already done great damage to the cause of law enforcement. Public officials will do well to disregard this unscientific, uncritical study and to regard marijuana as a menace wherever it is purveyed.

That the Federal Bureau of Narcotics and the *Journal of the American Medical Association* might have been overzealous and less than scientific and objective in their opinions is a factor that the drug's proponents insist must be taken into consideration. The latter group argue that, in testing the motor and sensory functions of the nervous system in regard to mental and physical deterioration due to cannabis, the La Guardia Report had selected its subjects on the basis of prolonged marijuana use. They were users accustomed to daily smoking for a period of up to sixteen years and they showed no abnormal systemic functioning that would differentiate them from the normal users.

The report also compared forty-eight users and twenty-four nonusers from the standpoint of mental and physical deterioration resulting from long-term use of marijuana and concluded that the smokers "had suffered no mental or physical deterioration as a result of their use of the drug." Another study by Friedman and Rockmore, "Marijuana: Factor in Personality Evaluation and Army Maladjustment," stated that their sample of 310 men who had used cannabis for an average of seven years showed no mental or physical deterioration.

However, the La Guardia Report did cite some deleterious effects of marijuana and explicitly concluded that under certain conditions it could cause psychotic reactions. In a few instances the anxiety experienced by the subject high on pot reached the panic level. In no cases, however, were there any acts of violence. As the effects of the drug wore off, the general sensation in most cases was one of drowsiness.

The report defines two types of psychotic reactions—an acute marijuana intoxication with a psychotic syndrome, and a state resembling a toxic psychosis. Acute intoxication is bound to follow any sufficiently large dose of marijuana, coming on promptly and passing off some hours later. In the marijuana-psychosis syndrome, the symptoms are much more severe and of longer duration. The report also mentioned several cases in which the psychotic state continued for a number of days and required hospitalization. It is not known which conditions predispose a person to the liability of a toxic psychosis although there is an indefinite duration factor involved. The relationship between the drug and the onset of a functional psychotic state is not always clear. The personality factor, however, is of undoubted importance and other toxic agents such as alcohol and other drugs as well as other metabolistic conditions may be involved.

The eleven cases the La Guardia Report investigators admitted to Bellevue Hospital illustrate the elusiveness of determining the dose considered psychotically toxic. The marijuana, taken in the form of cigarettes, was given to five Negroes and six whites, among them a Puerto Rican; one of the group was a homosexual, and all of them were of low intellectual and social order. The Puerto Rican soon became confused and excited, chasing people with an ice pick and showing distinct schizophrenic behavior.

Shortly after his discharge he was readmitted to the hospital, diagnosed as definitely psychotic, and transferred to a state hospital as a schizophrenic. The majority of the group—eight in fact—had psychopathic personalities previous to their involvement in the La Guardia experiments, and three of these were later transferred to state institutions for further care. This particular group studied by the La Guardia Report investigators were representative of those who come into contact with the police, and were then and now the kind of marijuana user who constitute the source of sensational newspaper and magazine stories.

In the main study itself, six of the subjects developed toxic episodes characteristic of acute marijuana intoxication. The dosage varied from four to eight cc. of concentrate and the episodes lasted from three to six hours, in one instance as long as ten hours. The doses were not toxic to others taking the same or even larger amounts. Once taken, the drug's effects were beyond the subject's control, resulting in abnormal behavior and disjointed speech. In three of the subjects a definite psychotic state occurred. Two showed symptoms immediately following marijuana ingestion; the third, after a two-week interval. One of the first pair was an epileptic and had a history of heroin addiction and a prepsychotic personality. The third was considered a case of prison psychosis. The conclusions were unanimous in that, with the potential personality makeup as well as the right time and environment, marijuana may bring on a true psychotic state.

It is important to note that none of the regular marijuana users included in the study were among the nine who had psychotic episodes. Four of the nine were occasional users while the other five were nonusers of marijuana. Although they received marijuana on several different occasions, the negative reactions were experienced during only one of their sessions.

In their studies *The Present Position of Hemp Drug Addiction in India* (1939), *The Use of Cannabis Drugs in India* (1957), and *Treatment of Drug Addiction: Experience in India* (1957), the Drs. Chopra collected detailed statistics on twelve hundred regular users in India, seventy percent of whom had practiced the habit for more than ten years. They found that seventy-two percent of those questioned used cannabis exclusively while the others also took alcohol, opium, or other drugs. The majority of those using the cannabis drink limited their intake to social occasions. Most investigators agree that generally no physiological dependence on marijuana is developed and only a slight tolerance is built up—a situation applying particularly to the moderate user in the United States.

Concerning cannabis use in India, the Drs. Chopra write: "The tolerance developed both in animals and man was generally slight, if any, and was in no way comparable to the tolerance developed to opiates. Its tolerance was observed only in those individuals who took excessive doses after prolonged use . . . Habitual use of *bhang* can be discontinued without much trouble." The study also showed that cannabis could be taken or left alone, observing that "many persons indulging in the *bhang* drink in summer discontinue it during the winter."

The La Guardia Report made exactly the same point in its study as to whether marijuana was addicting or not:

> A person may be a confined smoker for a prolonged period, and give up the drug voluntarily without experiencing any craving for it or exhibiting withdrawal symptoms. He may, at some time, later on, go back to its use. Others may remain infrequent users of the cigarette, taking one or two a week, or only when the "social setting" calls for participation.
>
> From time to time we had one of our investigators associate with a marihuana user. The investigator would bring up the subject of smoking. This would invariably lead to the suggestion that they obtain some marihuana cigarettes. They would seek a "tea pad," and if it was closed the smoker and our investigator would calmly resume their previous activity, such as the discussion of life in general or the playing of pool. There were apparently no signs indicative of frustration in the smoker at not being able to gratify the desire for the drug. We consider this point highly significant since it is so contrary to the experience of users of other narcotics.
>
> A similar situation occurring in one addicted to the use of morphine, cocaine, or heroin would result in a comprehensive attitude on the part of the addict to obtain the drug. If unable to secure it, there would be obvious physical and mental manifestations of frustration. This may be considered presumptive evidence that there is no true addiction in the medical sense associated with the use of marihuana.

Thus the sociological report of the La Guardia study yielded the following conclusions: "The practice of smoking marihuana does not lead to addiction in the medical sense of the word and the publicity concerning the catastrophic effects of marijuana smoking in New York City are unfounded."

The La Guardia Report researchers did not, however, limit themselves to the sociological data provided by their field investigators; they also carried out a clinical study of addiction and tolerance. They defined drug addiction as "characterized by a compelling urge to use the drug for the prevention or relief of distressing mental and physical disturbances which occur when the necessary dose is delayed or omitted. A drug habit is also characterized by an urge to use the drug, but this is not compelling. The abstinence symptoms, which are expressions of nervous state, are not particularly distressing and do not occur as long as the person's attention is placed on other matters. Drug tolerance, in the narrower sense used here, means that larger doses than were originally used are required to bring about the effects desired by the subject. In the case of morphine, tolerance develops because of addiction, but in other instances tolerance may be present without addiction and addiction without tolerance. When both are present, the matter takes on greater importance because of the extremes to which the addict goes to obtain the drug, constantly and in increasing quantities."

For their account of addiction and tolerance the La Guardia research group studied forty-eight users of marijuana. Most of this group claimed that they could and did voluntarily stop smoking for a time without any undue reaction caused by the deprivation.

The La Guardia Report concludes this particular study by saying: "The evidence available then—the absence of any compelling urge to use the drug, the absence of any distressing abstinence symptoms, the statement that no increase in dosage is required to repeat the desired effects in users—justifies the conclusion that neither true addiction nor tolerance is found in marihuana users. The continuation and the frequency of usage of marihuana, as in the case of many other habit-forming substances depends on the easily controlled desires for its pleasurable effects."

Corroborating the report's findings, Dr. Walter Bromberg, while director of the Psychiatric Clinic, Court of General Sessions in New York, stated: "The fact that offenders brought up on marijuana charges do not request medical treatment on their incarceration (with the cessation of drug supply) argues for the absence of withdrawal symptoms." Bromberg's article, "Marijuana, A Psychiatric Study," published in the *Journal of the American Medical Association* concluded from interviews with several hundred marijuana users that "true addiction was absent."

In 1967, the American Medical Association itself came around to a more charitable view in a release that concurred with the opinion that no physical dependence on marijuana has yet been demonstrated, that it has not been shown that marijuana causes addiction or leads to "any lasting mental or physical changes."

The confusion in the minds of the legislators about the connection between marijuana and the opiates revolves around their pet theory that the former leads inevitably to the latter. This idea has become so ingrained that the public has come to accept it as fact, although there is no conclusive evidence that tends to bear out this association. It is more probable that the indiscriminate binding together of the two types of drugs in the law books has made the connection between them more likely.

Legislative bias may derive some truth from the fact that the pusher who deals in both pot and heroin is often inclined to persuade the marijuana buyer to try some of his stronger opiates. Only the least-experienced smoker could possibly fall for this ploy since the knowledgeable marijuana user knows his preference and sticks by it. In America, particularly, the marijuana user is unfortunately more prone to come in contact with the pusher of both types of drugs than elsewhere, which accounts for the higher incidence of heroin abuse by former pot users even though there is neither a pharmacological nor physiological relation between the two drugs.

Federal narcotics agents, however, have always claimed that the marijuana user graduates to the more potent opiates in a natural quest for bigger kicks. The chief culprit in their eyes is the pusher, who is often suspected of being linked to the big crime syndicates controlling the heroin trade. This may be true, especially in the big cities, although today the shift of the pot phenomenon to the middle-class sector has had the result of relegating the criminal-type pusher to a far less prominent place than he once held. The connection for buying pot today is more likely to be an adventurous college student with little interest in pushing hard narcotics. Like the pot smoker, he is likely to be contemptuous of addicts "dumb" enough to fall for the "apple."

A now-defunct antinarcotics organization, the White Cross,

was extremely active in its portrayal of the pusher and his tricks. In a 1938 booklet, *On the Trial of Marihuana,* it depicted numerous innocents falling prey to the pusher and his bait. The organization claimed that the chain of evil, "the descent into hell," started with smoking ordinary cigarettes and subsequently it saw a direct link between the government-licensed tobacco companies and the peddler flogging his drugs. In their view, the stepping stones on the route to addiction led inevitably from tobacco to marijuana and thence to the opiates and the needle. It was never clarified just how this progression came about; it was accepted as fact and as such it was readily absorbed by the mass media and the public at large. Pot, they declared, might be the lesser of the drug evils, but it was the likely place for the occasional smoker on his way to permanent addiction to the opiates.

That this view is still current shows how well-entrenched this belief is in America. The press is constantly quoting law officials and "narks" whose statistics are accepted without question.

"Every user of heroin used marijuana first and then needed something stronger," says Westchester's Assistant District Attorney, T. A. Facelle (as quoted in the *New York Times*).

"A large majority of persons addicted to narcotic drugs have a history of marijuana use," claims Fred Dick of the Bureau of Narcotics in San Francisco.

An article in one of the last issues of the *Saturday Evening Post* cited a police estimate that thirty-seven percent of all addicts first turned on with marijuana, despite the contrary evidence supplied by the La Guardia Report and other studies.

One of the most influential studies to take sides with the general conclusions reached by the La Guardia Report was made by the Inter-Departmental Committee on Narcotics to President Eisenhower, which pointed out that "narcotic drugs differ from marijuana, which produces no physical dependence."

President Johnson's Crime Commission stated that "there are too many marijuana users that do not graduate to heroin, and too many heroin addicts with no known prior marijuana use, to support such a theory."

The latest evidence showing the tenuousness of the official position came with figures released in 1968 by Henry L. Giordano, former chief of the now-abolished FBN. According to Giordano, the number of known hard-drug addicts rose from

59,720 in 1966 to 62,045 by the end of 1967, a three-percent increase. As far as the bureau could determine, the number of new addicts increased from 6,047 to 6,417—a rise of such miniscule proportions that if only one in a hundred of the nation's marijuana users had switched to heroin last year, it would have shown in a far more dramatic increase in the number of newcomers to the heroin habit.

Addiction to opiates in the United States during the nineteenth and early part of the twentieth century often followed the abuse of alcohol, reports Dr. Alfred R. Lindesmith, professor of sociology at Indiana University. It still sometimes occurs in other parts of the world where it is known that morphine brings immediate relief to the alcoholic hangover. Morphine has been recommended as a cure for alcoholism, and at least one doctor deliberately addicted his alcoholic patients to this drug in the belief that it was the lesser of the two evils.

The stepping-stone theory of addiction has been pretty well discredited by the authoritative evidence now available; very few marijuana users go on to heroin. As Judge Charles Wyzanski stated in an article in the *Harvard Alumni Bulletin* in 1967: "It is, of course, absurd to argue that because most users of heroin first used marijuana, marijuana is proved to be a preliminary step to heroin addiction. One might as well say that because most users of heroin once imbibed milk, milk leads to heroin addiction." And an organ as conservative as the *Wall Street Journal* recently mentioned a twenty-two-year-old Harvard "nonhippie" who does smoke pot without any ill effects.

Dr. Lindesmith agrees that overt recommendation of marijuana use is not desirable. But he does point out that the disrepute in which it is held derives to a great extent from the drug's present "outlaw" status. He further indicates that just as a person under the influence of alcohol is not "himself," the individual "high" on pot is likely to act irresponsibly in such activities as driving an automobile or moving breakable wares. A comparison, however, between the aftereffects of marijuana and alcohol shows distinctly in favor of the drug, and Dr. Lindesmith concurs that alcohol constitutes a far greater social danger than does marijuana.

Even *Time,* which was once quick to pick up any tidbit substantiating the "Marijuana Menace," quotes a West Coast architect as saying that "pot certainly isn't addictive in the normal sense. For those who like it, it's as habit-forming as strawberry ice cream to people who love that dessert. Since my first try, I have gone as much as six months without so much as a puff." *Time* thus lends its considerable editorial power to the voices of reason in the marijuana controversy:

> Action in this direction [legalization] is obviously needed; like Prohibition's Volstead Act, current anti-marijuana laws only result in the arrest of increasing thousands of young Americans each year without any deterrent effect. The use of marijuana is thus becoming a social phenomena rather than a legal nuisance, but medical science and the law have not kept up with the change.

As this book goes to press, there are almost daily headlines on the new "Marijuana Menace." On February 2, 1969, the *New York Times* released a report containing new and alarming data collected by Dr. William F. Geber, a pharmacologist at the University of Georgia who has been studying possible links between marijuana and birth defects in animals. Although he concedes that his experiments furnish little solid knowledge about the drug's related effects on man, his findings are, as he puts it, "enough . . . to give us a real scare."

Dr. Geber revealed that marijuana, like LSD, may affect the development of fetuses and the genetic characteristics of organisms. When Geber injected large doses of the cannabis resin into pregnant rabbits and hamsters, they developed dead or malformed fetuses, with special injury to the brain, spine, limbs, and liver. Further, some of the fetuses were abnormally small. The malformations, he pointed out, appeared to be closely related to the dosages of marijuana, for control animals injected with a saline solution produced litters without such defects.

At peak dosages, rabbits showed only a tiny fraction of the group unaffected: Sixty-nine percent of the fetuses were reabsorbed; thirteen percent of those issued were dead; and two-thirds of those born alive were either malformed or runted. Hamsters that received similarly high dosages showed much less damage. At low dosages both groups were unaffected. His results, Geber warns, show how little we actually know about marijuana.

A more recent article in the March 10, 1969, issue of the *New York Times* entitled "Drug Use Rises in City's High Schools" suggested that there may be a shift in the present scene because of the markedly soaring rate with which the middle class has taken to indulgence in drugs, especially marijuana.

The article gave estimates of marijuana use ranging from thirty to eighty percent of some student bodies and stated that it can be found in virtually all New York City secondary schools —not only in the overcrowded public institutions but in the exclusive private ones as well. The author found that pot smoking seems to have "no ethnic boundaries" and has spread rapidly throughout middle- and upper-class student bodies. Age boundaries are slipping away, too, according to the article, which reported the findings of a San Francisco sociologist who had discovered fifth-graders in California smoking marijuana.

The use of marijuana by increasing numbers of teen-agers and even younger groups frightens authorities for good reason. These new young drug users have a casual and apparently fearless attitude toward drugs. In their ignorance, they may heedlessly experiment with the more dangerous chemicals. The *New York Times* did, in fact, reveal an open and growing use of heroin, cocaine, LSD, and amphetamines in some advantaged areas. If students purchase pot and heroin from the same source, they may well assume that one is no more dangerous than the other.

Although most pot smokers generally stick to marijuana, and as the *Times* article declared, most students "distinguish quite carefully between the drugs and the types of users. . .and classify marijuana with cigarettes and alcohol, not with such potent drugs as heroin or LSD," not all of them are so discriminating and knowledgeable. With the amazingly low age groups using pot, the danger is doubly increased, for it can hardly be expected that twelve- or thirteen-year-olds will be aware of the finer points of addiction. Although it is true that pot smokers in college and hippie communities (from middle-class backgrounds and probably cognizant of the properties of the various drugs, especially the perils of heroin) tend to avoid the hard drugs, this cannot be said for their ghetto counterparts. The *Times* report found that "heroin and other narcotics are used mostly by low-income Negro and Puerto Rican students." The other students, if they use drugs other than marijuana, favor LSD or other hallucinogens.

Nevertheless, according to reliable reports, a growing number of youngsters from affluent areas have been moving from marijuana to heroin. While the Negro and Puerto Rican students are under stronger pressure in this respect because they live in areas where heroin addiction is an adult problem, the advantaged students to whom pot is a cheap, easy escape from school boredom may find the more potent drugs a temptation (although those who do advance to more dangerous drugs are generally plagued by psychological problems).

The gravity of the entire drug situation is pointed up by Dr. Donald Louria who, as president of the New York State Council on Drug Addiction, states that "the use of heroin among white kids was just not around two years ago. Now it is getting to be an alarming problem." He goes on to express concern at the mounting number of teen-agers who are taking various combinations of drugs—sometimes with tragic results.

Thus, although the percentage of marijuana users who go on to heroin (including ghetto residents) is still relatively small, the huge increase of total marijuana smokers, which now contains a good section of the middle class, results in a greater number of individuals who might become addicted to hard harcotics.

So we see that a relationship between marijuana and heroin does exist. But it is not the simple, causal step-by-step theory outlined earlier. It is a far more complex one.

The *New York Times* evaluated the legalization of marijuana in terms of removing it from its underworld connection to heroin. Has the common approach toward these two disparate drugs contributed to the problem? An illustration of the dangers of this attitude was given wherein a dealer pawned off an opiate as something else by tagging it with an exotic name.

Some authorities favor placing heroin addicts on a medical treatment plan that permits addicts to purchase their necessary doses legally. This approach, they point out, would relieve heroin users of the need to "push" narcotics that trap others in the opiate web. It would also "break the back" of the Mafia-controlled heroin racket. Many of the same people propose a controlled legal outlet for marijuana to take its sales away from illegal sellers.

Other experts, however, believe the easy accessibility of pot would only result in a much larger number of marijuana consumers. This new following, they insist, would swell the count of smokers destined to go on to hard narcotics.

The advocates of legalization rebut that argument by contending that legalization of pot and the removal of all the myths surrounding it, along with a program of education dealing with the dangers of the narcotics, would most likely have the beneficial effect of turning many people away from such drugs as heroin. In addition, it could be expected to create a more humane atmosphere for the treatment and possible cure of the addict.

Indeed, as Dr. Geber told the *Times,* "This is a forest we've been dropped into. We're either in the middle of it or on the periphery of it and it's night. It might take five minutes or three years to get out of it."

CHAPTER SEVEN

POT AND THE ESTABLISHMENT: THE SOCIAL ASPECTS

Crime, Sex, Cigarettes, Autos, and Alcohol

The irony underlying much of the official view on marijuana is that knowledgeable spokesmen consider it less dangerous than those indispensable extensions of life in America—automobiles, alcohol, and cigarettes. Four decades of repressive measures have reinforced the imaginary links between the drug and violent crimes, sexual depravities, and even madness. The following statement by Henry L. Giordano, the former Commissioner of the now-defunct Bureau of Narcotics, is representative of the "official" view held by police departments across the country:

> From my studies and experience, one theme emerges—that marijuana is capable of inducting acts of violence, even murder. The drug frees the unconscious tendencies of the individual user, the result being reflected in frequent quarrels, fights and assaults. (For example) in Colorado, a man under the influence of marijuana attempted to kill his wife, but killed her grandmother instead, and then committed suicide . . . In Oriental countries . . . there exist stupefied wretches, who are a danger and a burden to their society because of marijuana use . . . Even Patrice Lumumba was known to authorities as an habitual user of marijuana and this was believed to have contributed to his irrational behavior.

Such statements, portraying the marijuana user as a pitiful being stalking the fringes of society like an automaton devoid of any power to change his course, are countless. A weak, amoral person, he must be hunted down and isolated so as not to contaminate the simon-pure complexion of his environment, according to the law enforcers. They are unanimous that he is a threat to all established values, even though today's pot smoker is usually a college student or professional well above the average intellectual mean.

This is not to say that the record of marijuana users is one-hundred-percent pure. Certainly marijuana may have been involved in situations of orgiastic abandonment—just as alcohol and stag movies may spark off equally inflammable conduct. Violent crimes are occasionally committed by corporation executives, society debs, honor students, hardened criminals, and marijuana smokers. Intellectual honesty forbids putting the blame solely at the door of the pad where marijuana is smoked.

The opposite argument that marijuana is the universal panacea, the magic drug capable of changing the whole world into an idyllic turned-on place, is equally fallacious.

"If only all the government leaders would smoke pot, the world would be an infinitely better place," is a sentiment often voiced by starry-eyed smokers, overwhelmed by the drug's soothing influence.

There is no denying that it does tend to have a calming effect on people—far more than alcohol—and is especially suited for those of a contemplative turn of mind. On the other hand, marijuana is not a miracle worker. It cannot make genius out of a common mind and does not inspire the mediocre to brilliance. Its magic is limited to raising the consciousness to a sometimes sharper awareness, but it cannot effect a wholesale transformation of the personality in question.

As Dr. Howard S. Becker, the professor of sociology at Northwestern University who was the first American sociologist to explain the sociological implications of marijuana, has stated, "Marijuana does not change the basic personality structure of an individual. It lessens inhibitions and this brings out what is latent in the user's thoughts, but does not evoke responses which would otherwise be totally alien to him."

In this chapter we shall examine the allegations leveled against marijuana—its supposed criminal and aphrodisiac effects, as well as the motivating force underlying the cultural taboo that has been placed upon it.

The marijuana myths of the twenties and thirties linger on. Propaganda about the "inherent evils" of marijuana is aired over and over again in public documents. "The Narcotic Problem: A Brief Study—1965" by the California Bureau of Narcotic Enforcement is typical. It states:

> Its greatest dangers are that the intoxication and hallucinations produced may lead to violent conduct, such as attacking a friend, thinking that it is necessary for self-defense. . . . The user of marijuana is a dangerous individual and should definitely not be underestimated by police officers . . . known users of either cocaine or marijuana . . . may be dangerous, hard to handle, and might resort to any act of violence.

Despite such prophecies of doom, the numerous studies investigating the alleged connection between marijuana and crime are almost all unanimous in their agreement that no such link exists. The precedent for the association between crime and pot dates as far back as 650 years ago to Marco Polo's description of how cannabis was used by Hasan and his band of assassins. We have observed how in the United States near-hysteria developed about 1930 when the use of marijuana was related to a violent crime wave and the widespread corruption of schoolchildren.

Dr. Frank R. Gomila, Commissioner of Public Safety in New Orleans at the time, wrote that some homes for boys were "full of children who had become habituated to the use of cannabis," and of the mindless crimes committed by the "youngsters known as 'muggleheads,' " fortified by the narcotic. Some sixty-eight percent of the crimes committed in New Orleans in 1936 were attributed to marijuana users.

Despite these lurid claims, subsequent studies have, for the most part, failed to establish a direct link between major crime and cannabis. The La Guardia Report found that some marijuana smokers were guilty of petty offenses, but again there was no evidence showing the drug to be at the root of these crimes. It was considered far more likely that the smokers were simply petty criminals who happened to use pot. The report indicated a complete lack of substantiation for marijuana's alleged association with major crime.

More recent assessments tend to agree with these findings. *The Ad Hoc Panel on Drug Abuse* at the 1962 White House Conference states: "Although marijuana has long held the reputation of inciting individuals to commit sexual offenses and other antisocial acts, evidence is inadequate to substantiate this."

In many countries alcohol is considered to be far more of a threat to public order than cannabis. According to an editorial in the *South African Medical Journal, "Dagga* (a South African preparation of cannabis) produces in the smoker drowsiness, euphoria, and occasional psychotic episodes, but alcohol is guilty of even graver action. It is not certain to what extent *dagga* contributes to the commission of crime in this country. Alcohol does so in undeniable measure."

In this country, Dr. Walter Bromberg, as psychiatrist in charge of the Psychiatric Clinic of the Court of General Sessions in New York, conducted two full-scale statistical studies on marijuana smoking and the incidence of crimes of violence in the city. The results of the first of these studies were presented at the 89th Annual Meeting of the American Psychiatric Association. He stated that in a two-year survey of over two thousand felonies not one case of marijuana smoking was discovered. None of the assaults or sex crimes committed were due to marijuana intoxication. Bromberg made it clear that his study also showed no direct correspondence between violent crime and marijuana.

His second report, "Marijuana: A Psychiatric Study," was published in the *Journal of the American Medical Association:*

> Sporadic reports of murders and assaults due to marijuana appear in the press frequently. It is difficult to evaluate these statements, because of their uncritical nature. The bulletin prepared by the Foreign Policy Association lists ten cases "culled at random from the files of the U.S. Bureau of Narcotics" of murder and atrocious assault in which marijuana was directly responsible for the crime. Among the ten patients, the second, J.O., was described as having confessed how he murdered a friend and put his body in a trunk while under the influence of marijuana.
>
> J.O. was examined in this clinic; although he was a psychopathic liar and possibly homosexual, there was no indication in the examination or history of the use of any drug. The investigation by the probation department failed to indicate use of the drug marijuana. The deceased, however, was addicted to heroin.

Admitting the difficulty in obtaining objective statements on the marijuana experience of some seventeen thousand prisoners interviewed over a six-and-a-half-year period, Bromberg nevertheless found several hundred pot smokers whose evidence invariably squared with the experimental and clinical tests previously carried out. He noted the same symptoms of intoxication observed in the clinical experiments, as well as a lack of true addiction and an absence of any substantive connection with major crimes, such as sexual assault and murder.

On the basis of a concommitant study of drug offenders convicted by the New York County Court of Special Sessions, Bromberg estimated that a total of 540, or nine percent of all drug offenders coming before the court, were users of marijuana. Observes Bromberg: "Among those with longer records, that is, from four to seven arrests, none showed progression from the use of drugs to other crimes."

He concludes that as a result of these findings, it "can be said that drugs generally do not initiate criminal careers," although he admits as "a matter of speculation" whether the first offenders indicted on marijuana use go on to major crime. The expectancy of this in New York County is small, according to Bromberg.

Another study, conducted by the La Guardia Report investigators, limited itself to the relationship between marijuana and juvenile delinquency. Although they registered the evidence as negative, today's school grounds, especially in overcrowded ghetto areas, are not the same as they were twenty-five years ago at the time the report was made. Not only did the field investigators then find little evidence of marijuana use in New York City high schools, they also failed to produce proof of a tendency toward juvenile delinquency due to the small incidence of pot smoking that did occur at the time. The picture has changed in the quarter-century since. The rising statistics of juvenile crime and the popularity of pot among high-school students today seem to establish a more definite link between the two. The La Guardia Report confirms that marijuana smoking could be an incidental, but rarely a contributory, cause of crime. The sociological conditions of our times have given an impetus to both crime and the use of marijuana, whose common denominator is a disregard for law and authority. Apart from this shared characteristic, the two activities seem to have developed in parallel, rather than interconnecting lines.

It also observed that "in marijuana literature the action of the drug is usually described from retrospective observation of the effect on a single individual. Relationship to varying dosage, to the subject's varying personality and background, to environmental conditions when the drug was taken, is given little, if any, attention. It is the lack of information concerning these and other factors involved in marijuana reaction which has given rise to the present confusion regarding its effects."

The report concluded that in those cases where an individual smoked marijuana and engaged in crime, the criminality came first and not the other way around, although this is questioned by United States and state law-enforcement agencies. Former FBN Commissioner Giordano speaks for many of his colleagues when he describes the use of marijuana as "a vice which draws with it a train of depravities stretching far into the future."

In 1967, Dr. Sanford Feinglass of the University of California Medical School elaborated on the disinhibiting effects of marijuana. His conclusion is that even if marijuana does release inhibitions, "it is not certain that the user will be moved to act." The effect of marijuana on behavior, Feinglass and some other investigators believe, depends more on the individual's own natural inclinations than on any sinister property residing in the drug.

Similarly, Dr. H. B. Murphy of McGill University writes in "The Cannabis Habit: A Review of Recent Psychiatric Literature," published in the *Bulletin of Narcotics*: "Most serious observers agree that cannabis does not, per se, induce aggressive or criminal activity, in that the reduction of the work drive leads to a negative correlation with criminality rather than a positive one."

The drug, he points out, may release repressed feelings of hostility, but alcohol, he adds, will do the same. But careful study would indicate that one is much more likely to act under the influence of alcohol than under the calming influence of marijuana. From observations of marijuana smokers it is difficult to see how the intoxicated individual could motivate himself adequately to go through the motions of a crime. Such a simple act as getting a lighter to work or pouring a glass of water not infrequently become laborious exercises under the drug's influence, and one may often find a person high on pot in a complete state of confusion when it comes to performing the most trivial routines of daily life.

How then did marijuana receive its reputation as a decisive factor in the incidence of crime? The police may be partly blamed for their readiness to accept this belief as an a priori fact—an idea that colors their approach to crime and their manner of handling it. Another contributing factor may be their experience with a highly select sample of marijuana users. Rarely, if ever, do they come into contact with the executives, and lawyers, who smoke pot. At the same time, they have no firsthand knowledge of the effects of marijuana. Although this may not necessarily restrict the efficiency of their operations, it does limit it.

Newspaper accounts are perhaps the biggest source of misinformation concerning the drug because of the emphasis on the kind of story that makes good "copy." The more sensational the details and the more bizarre the behavior, the greater the likelihood of the story appearing in print. Since the real facts behind marijuana use are too pedestrian to be reported, the stories that do appear reflect the bias of the official view because they are based largely on police reports.

Equally influential is the fact that marijuana can be obtained only in an illegal manner. According to the statutes, both buying and growing the hemp plant are reprehensible and any purchaser would have to deal of necessity with a connection who, by this very activity, is violating the law. The pusher is considered a criminal, and so are his associates. Smoking pot is a crime, keeping it in the home is a crime, and giving it away is a crime. As soon as an individual exchanges any money for the purchase of marijuana or has it in his possession, he is marked as a criminal.

It is not surprising, therefore, that the pot smoker comes to look at the law with a different eye—it is no longer a protective agent but something to be shunned. Like every other criminal, he begins to inhabit a shadow world where every policeman is a threat and every strange knock at the door is suspect.

Dr. Howard S. Becker, who has been described earlier as the first American sociologist to delve accurately into the motivations of people using marijuana, explains the attitude developed by the pot smoker:

> Marijuana use illustrates the way deviant motives actually develop in the course of experience with the deviant activity. To put a complex argument in a few words: Instead of the deviant motives leading to the deviant behavior, it is the other way around; the deviant behavior in crime produces the deviant motivation. Vague impulses and desires—in this case, probably

most frequently a curiosity about the kind of experience the drug will produce—are transformed into definite patterns of action.

A good deal of this "curiosity" stems from an unspoken belief that marijuana opens the doors to exhilarating sex experiences that are different and far more ecstatic than the ordinary. Marijuana is considered the seed of uncontrollable sex urges—an aphrodisiac similar in its effect to cantharides but minus the latter's concommitant risks. Authoritative opinion hews to two conflicting views, as shown in the following accounts from "Two Cases of Cannabis Indica Intoxication" in the *Therapeutic Gazette* of two different witnesses describing the same effect.

One experimenter with the drug reports on his experience with marijuana after an initial period of anxiety: ". . . then of all the happy mortals that ever existed, I was the most supremely so. I saw the most beatific visions, the most beautiful women, angelic in their mental and physical configurations. If all the gold of Solomon's Temple had been offered to me, I would not then have relinquished my perfect happiness and mutual repose."

On the other hand, C. W. Burr, the author of the essay, says that during his experience "sex ideas were entirely absent and Venus herself could not have tempted me."

Richard Burton, translater of the *Arabian Nights,* claimed that it was used in the Orient to prolong coition as well as to increase the intensity of the sensation.

This belief was echoed by Hector France: "Hashish is, of course, a positive aphrodisiac, the length of the venereal act being at one reinforced and repeated."

Indian and Chinese books on the art of love extol hemp as a restorer and invigorator of sexual power and they have long been known in houses of ill repute as stimulants to stir flagging sexual prowess. However, it is curious to note that Indian monks and recluses use hemp to suppress their sexual desires in their renunciation of worldly pleasures.

In the Indian study conducted by the Drs. Chopra, a sample of some twelve thousand people found ten percent listing sexual factors as a reason for indulging in the cannabis habit. They write, "Amongst profligate women and prostitutes, *bhang* sherbet used to be a popular drink in the course of an evening when their paramours visited them. This practice has, however, been largely replaced by the drinking of alcohol, which is much more harmful." The two investigators also mentioned the "saintly people who wish to renounce worldly pleasure and use cannabis drugs for suppressing their sexual desires."

In North Africa it is widely believed that cannabis will preserve, maintain, or improve sexual powers, while in the United States, H. C. Wood, one of the first American students of the drug, found that "at no time were there any aphrodisiac feelings produced." But a co-worker of his, after taking a preparation of the drug, not only became ravenously hungry but also found himself roused to a state of "veneral excitement" accompanied by priapism that lasted for several days.

Dr. R. P. Walton did not think of the drug itself as an aphrodisiac but believed that it could produce this result through exerting a paralytic action on the higher structures of the brain and thereby releasing the lower, more primitive structures that are normally restrained and controlled by the cerebral cortex.

This view concurs with those of Drs. Samuel Allentuck and Karl Bowman: "Marijuana is no more aphrodisiac than is alcohol. Unlike damiana, yohimbin, testosterone propionate, etc., which produced genitial engorgement directly, marijuana like alcohol, acts only indirectly through the cerebral cortex in this respect."

Thorvald T. Brown, a former detective, corroborated these clinical findings in his book, *The Enigma of Drug Addiction,* published by C. C. Thomas in 1961:

> Tales out of the past to the contrary, marijuana does not act as an aphrodisiac. Smokers, both male and female, have indicated that they experience no change in libido as a result of the drug and do not associate it with sex . . . The so-called sex parties at which marijuana is smoked are often reported in the press as though marijuana was the cause of these orgies. Again, the drug does no more than relax the inhibitions and the promiscuity which may result could just as likely result from over-indulgence in alcohol at a cocktail party.

It is not unreasonable to conclude, therefore, that if the person is sexually oriented and has sex on his mind, the inhibition-releasing effect of marijuana could lead him to a desire for congress or the activity itself. Since an overdose of marijuana tends to produce a narcotic or soporific effect, it would be an unlikely stimulant to sexual prowess as expressed in acts of congress.

Furthermore, although coition may be a more intense experience under the influence of marijuana, it is still an activity that takes place apart from the drug itself.

For instance, a person with his mind set on painting may derive greater enjoyment from it while high than if he were doing it while sober. In other words, as noted in the examples given of smokers in India, where marijuana is used both as a sexual stimulant and repressant, the drug's effects are subject to the user's suggestibility—its effects parallel his convictions as to what it will do to him, and the feelings he derives come from none other but himself.

Sexual aggressiveness, according to Dr. Richard Blum of Stanford's Institute for the Study of Human Problems, operates independently from marijuana's properties. Despite the persistent reports that it may act to intensify sexual pleasure—for example, by prolonging orgasm—Blum doesn't consider the drug an aphrodisiac.

The erotic effects of marijuana were also examined by the La Guardia Report investigation in a clinical study carried out on volunteers in the more objective surroundings of the hospital. Only in about ten percent of the one hundred and fifty instances in which marijuana was administered to the specific group did the findings give evidence of eroticism, even during psychotic episodes. In one isolated instance there was a case of frank exhibitionism, but the investigators did not relate the cause to marijuana; the subject, who was not a regular marijuana user, had been arrested on three occasions for similar instances of indecent exposure.

Thus it is readily observable that marijuana does not, by itself, induce uncontrollable sexual urges in the smoker. Virtually all investigators agree that the possible aphrodisiac qualities of cannabis are cerebral in nature and stem from the reduction of inhibitions and increased suggestibility. It is probable that it is little, if any more, effective than alcohol in this respect, which brings us to the questions of alcohol and cigarettes—the "approved" drugs of the American way of life.

No opprobrium attaches to the two-pack-a-day smoker, and few would raise an eyebrow at the executive who goes through his day with a two-martini lunch and a few drinks before and after dinner. Our cigarettes come in convenient packages and, despite the warning printed boldly on the container that "cigarette smoking may be hazardous to your health," we continue to inhale a veritable chimney stack of nicotine fumes each day.

It is popular knowledge that tobacco smoking may result in the growth of cancerous malignancies, destruction of lung cells, heart disease, and a shortening of the actual life span by a good many years. Yet, the fact that we have developed a physiological dependence on, if not a mild physical addiction to, cigarettes is considered hardly alarming enough to be worthy of comment. The effort to quit smoking, as anyone knows who has tried it, is an ordeal demanding a concentration of will power and self discipline few of us can muster.

We are all familiar with the irritable, nervous person in the midst of quitting his tobacco habit and we readily condone his condition, knowing the agony of the withdrawal symptoms he is suffering. At the same time it is hard to imagine an actual ban being placed upon the sale and consumption of cigarettes.

"With forty percent of the population smoking," says United States Surgeon General Dr. William M. Stuart, "I don't think the public would stand up for a ban. We had one experience with prohibition and I think it would, based on that experience, have the same kind of result."

We similarly poison the body with alcohol—a brew that not only wreaks havoc on the stomach and liver but that can actually destroy these organs. Overindulgence robs the body of essential vitamins, and may even produce insanity. The hangover following a drinking bout is a physically debilitating condition in which little is remembered of the previous night. Alcohol is often a factor in a violent crime, and drunken drivers are responsible for countless tragedies on America's highways. Prohibition, instead of relieving the problems caused by alcohol, aggravated them because people were simply unwilling to give up their intoxicants. Today drinking is a respectable social indulgence, and the person who can hold his liquor is admired for his capacity.

Tobacco and alcohol are legal and easily accessible to adults; they support two sizeable industries, and are touted in newspaper ads and billboards across the country. Marijuana, on the other hand, presents a different picture. It has been denounced for producing exhilaration, loss of inhibitions, a changed sense of time, and other psychological effects—effects of intoxication.

Dr. Alfred R. Lindesmith, professor of sociology at Indiana

University, has stated categorically that "Intrinsically marijuana is less dangerous and harmful to the human body than is alcohol." He goes on to point out:

> Ironically, the accusations that are leveled at marijuana are all applicable to alcohol, as has been demonstrated by innumerable investigations. These studies indicate that much murder, rape, and homicide are committed by persons under the influence. The special psychoses and ailments of alcoholics are numerous and well-delineated in countless scientific and literary productions. The menace of the drinking driver of automobiles is well-understood by all and is more or less accepted as one of the inevitable hazards of life in the modern world.
>
> It is well-known, too, that the manufacturers of alcoholic beverages advertise their products and seek to enlarge their markets, and that the use of alcohol spreads from those who already have the practice to those who do not. Why, then, so much excitement about marijuana? It is said that marijuana sometimes causes girls and women to lose their virtue and innocence, but the role of alcohol in this respect is infinitely more important. It seems inconsistent, therefore, that while the decision to drink or not to drink is viewed as a personal moral decision, the use of marijuana should be viewed as a heinous crime subject to long prison sentences.*

Dr. Joel Fort, who has served on the medical staff of the Federal Narcotics Hospital in Lexington, Kentucky, and as consultant on drug addiction to the World Health Organization, in addition to having been a lecturer in the School of Criminology at the University of California at Berkeley and Director of the Center for Treatment and Education on Alcoholism in Oakland, California, has some pertinent observations on the subject:

> If marijuana were not called terrible by society, everyone would find it a mild drug that has little effect except to stimulate the appetite, slow down the time sense and create a mild euphoria, and that would be that. In the countries where it is widely used, there is no scientific proof of overall harm or danger to the individual or to society. Marijuana might well be more beneficial to mankind than alcohol, but any reform of present laws would probably be opposed by the alcoholic beverage industry and cer-

*From *The Addict and the Law* by Alfred Lindesmith. Copyright © Indiana University Press. Reprinted by permission.

tainly by poorly informed legislators and representatives of law enforcement.

The La Guardia Report also surveyed this aspect of marijuana. In order to observe the sociological effects the drug might have on the "American way of life," the investigators carried out extensive tests on the hospital volunteers, examining their moral, family, and community ideologies to see if they would be affected by marijuana use.

They found, in general, that the subject's attitude toward family and community ties, as manifested in the evidence of the research, did not change markedly as the result of pot smoking. In fact, the only such change was in his attitude toward the drug itself. Before trying marijuana only four of fourteen subjects said they would tolerate the sale of marijuana, while after ingestion, eight of them pronounced themselves in favor of it. In other words, by experiencing the drug they became aware that it was not as bad as they had heard it would be.

Similarly, the recent rise in pot smoking as a recreational device can be attributed to the credibility gap between the generations. Pot smokers, and others who have been exposed to the practice, now scoff at the old tales of depravity, crime, addiction, and promiscuity that they were warned would inevitably follow the first "toke" of marijuana.

Dr. David Smith, the head of San Francisco General Hospital's Alcohol and Drug Screening Unit, who has come into contact with many of the Haight-Ashbury marijuana users, is agitated by the marijuana credibility gap. He asks the parents of the youngsters he encounters, "How can you expect your children to respect authorities who will ruin a person's life for possession of marijuana and put a man in jail for using a drug with the abuse potential of a cocktail? Police tell young people that smoking pot will turn them into addicts. They know it's not true."

There is, according to student pot smokers, a general hypocrisy in America regarding the use of drugs. They claim that the same society that now punishes the pot smoker with lengthy imprisonment for use of a mild hallucinogen is itself most guilty of reckless indulgence in pharmaceutical drugs and other stimulants. The person who condemns pot inhales his first morning nicotine as soon as he wakes up; he follows this up by a dose of caffeine; by noon he has consumed half a pack of cigarettes; during lunch he downs two shots of alcohol, has another martini when he comes home, downs some more caffeine after dinner, takes a pill to go to sleep and a tranquilizer to smooth out his nerves so that he'll be able to function better at the office or on the golf course.

The fight over marijuana is part of a running battle between the mainstream of American society and an alienated minority under thirty. For many in this new generation, marijuana has become a flag of discontent to wave in the face of traditional American values. The division between the age groups has been described by folk singer Judy Collins as a conflict between the "marijuana generation" and the "alcohol generation." To youngsters today, pot is their symbol of emancipation from traditional values—a thing completely their own, untarnished by an adult society they distrust.

"The older generation," says Father Carlo Weber, a Jesuit priest and psychologist at Los Angeles's Loyola University, "lives in an achievement culture, zeroed in on alcohol as symbolized by the cocktail party where people go to become anonymous and dip into a great cloud of escape. The new generation doesn't want to run away. It wants to look at the ultimates."

University of California's sociologist E. Z. Friedenberg, author of *The Vanishing Adolescent,* adds: "Alcohol primarily relieves anxiety and promotes optimism. It makes the society and what one has to do with society okay. Pot, on the other hand, turns you inside yourself. Imagine a twenty-fifth college reunion with pot, not flasks."

It has been alleged that this country's drug laws bear the imprint of an attempt to legislative morality under the guise of preventing violent criminal acts. Laws generally are instituted to direct the morality and values that reflect the will of a majority of its members. But in the case of the drug laws, the result has been to impose confusion rather than order. There is a definite cleavage between their intent and the explanation of why they exist. Withdrawal into the limbo of the altered consciousness is anathema to the achievement-oriented Western society, and indulgence in cannabis is often followed by a new and different conception of our competitive and aggressive world.

G. M. Carstairs, in his study, "Cultural Factors in Choice of Intoxicants," noted in India that a basic difference in cultural values underlies the choice of alcohol by the aggressive Rajputs and cannabis by the more passive Brahmins. Most primitive cultures choose alcohol in that it releases aggressive action, while cannabis is associated with a characteristic sense of euphoria, which is likely to lead to a more passive personality with prolonged regular use.

H. B. M. Murphy, professor of psychology at McGill University, follows a similar line of reasoning as to why cannabis is banned in the West while alcohol is not only permitted but also carries a seal of social approval. In his essay, "The Cannabis Habit," he writes:

> In Anglo-Saxon cultures inaction is looked down on and often feared, whereas overactivity, aided by alcohol or independent of alcohol, is considerably tolerated despite the social disturbance produced. It may be that we can ban cannabis simply because the people who use it, or would do so, carry little weight in social matters and are relatively easy to control; whereas the alcohol user often carries plenty of weight in social matters and is difficult to control, as the United States Prohibition era showed. It has yet to be shown, however, that the one is more socially or personally disruptive than the other.

This concurs with the fact that only in the past few years has marijuana use in this country spread from the less achievement-oriented minority groups to the more career-minded middle classes. All at once, the dominant alcohol-using culture can be seen shifting its preferences to marijuana through the vanguard of a younger generation expressing its discontent with a materialistic, competitive society. The current hippie subculture has proclaimed vociferously that it refuses to walk the road trod by its elders, and has chosen marijuana and other hallucinogenics rather than alcohol as a guide to a more meaningful life.

Alienation and discontent with life in America is not felt by the younger generation alone. Responsible members of the government and communities across the country are aware of the dehumanizing tendencies in our increasingly technology-oriented society. It is significant that the hippie movement—mainly a white middle-class movement—has penetrated their consciousness to an extent never reached when the use of drugs was chiefly limited to minority groups, specifically the Negro subculture. With the puritanical ethic giving ground to a view in which pleasure for its own sake is considered a valid experience, the emphasis on life in America today is shifting to an exploration of inward rather than community-based values.

An interesting fact about the history of drugs in North America, and one which should give comfort to those concerned about the present trend, is that the stronger hallucinogens have been known in the United States for a longer period than marijuana. At the turn of the century, a vociferous outcry was raised over the spread of peyote and mescaline, yet in the sixty years since the holocaust of moral degeneration predicted by the alarmists has not materialized. According to some authorities, it is from this basis that present laws should take their direction, since it should be clear by now that continued repression is not likely to dispel the tide of pot fumes now washing over America.

William H. McGlothlin, whose essay *Toward a Rational View of Marijuana* appears in *Marijuana: Myths And Realities,* published by Brandon House in 1967, lists the reasons advanced by proponents of legislation. These advocates, he writes:

> . . . contend that it falls within an individual's constitutional rights; that a person should be permitted to use chemical as well as other means of consciousness alteration in the pursuit of religious experience, self-understanding, and even pleasure. Specifically, they contend that prohibition violates the First Amendment's guarantee of freedom of religion, and more generally, that it is an unwarranted invasion of privacy . . . the basic right to be let alone, as set forth by the Fourteenth Amendment. They argue further that any harmful effects are confined to the individual, society not suffering directly, and that legal attempts to protect an individual from himself are basically unworkable. The issue is one of prohibition and not regulation; the constitutional right of the government to regulate drugs in the public interest is not questioned.
>
> The opposing viewpoint holds that the concept of individual freedom is by no means absolute and the very fact that a government exists entails individual restraints in the interest of the public good . . . that harmful effects of drug use are not confined to the individual, but indirectly affect society in a variety of ways. While the arguments of prohibiting marijuana on the grounds that it causes crime and leads to heroin have been shown to be fallacious, more valid arguments might be made that its use could lead to a less productive economy, or that a nation of marijuana

and LSD users would be more vulnerable to attack from outside aggressors.

Considering marijuana and the stronger hallucinogens together, the question could be asked as to whether, or when, the state has a right to protect itself against a chemical assault on its value system, a threat that might, if sufficiently widespread, endanger the present social order.

It is likely that the seesaw of arguments pro and con will rock for some time to come. The drug question involves a whole value system. The legalization of marijuana and other drugs would constitute a radically new departure from traditional patterns for which the public must be prepared in advance.

CHAPTER EIGHT

POT AND THE AUTHORITIES: THE LEGISLATION

From the Marijuana Menace to LeMar

In the West the legal battle against marijuana began when Napoleon invaded Egypt at the end of the eighteenth century and attempted, unsuccessfully, to outlaw the hashish dens he found there. He bore down hard on the marijuana traffic by meting out severe punishments to violators, but the drug remained available in France throughout his rule. Commerce between France and the Middle East made hashish easily accessible and its use spread among a number of avant-garde writers and intellectuals.

In frontier America, coffee, alcohol, and tobacco were the few drugs permitted by a sober-living society. There was no drug "problem" in the United States until after the Civil War when American society began to undergo a number of rapid changes. The first drug to gain wide currency was opium, although it was neither smoked openly as it was in the Orient, nor surreptitiously as in the opium dens of the Middle East after the Europeans there had forced it underground.

For a time it became one of the most widely used drugs in America. In the form of paregoric (a tincture of opium), it was available under such brand names as Sergeant Williams' Health Giving Elixir, Uncle Chollie's Effluvious Spring Tonic, Indian Joe's Miracle Medicine, The Friendly Brothers' Cure-All Water, Fields' Fabulous Fluid, Stratford's Syrup, Powell's Proper Power-Potion, Colonel Nimrod's Miracle Syrup, and a thousand other potions that promised cures for everything from warts and rickets to the plague. In those days any patent medicine purchased at the neighborhood pharmacy was likely to contain a good percentage of opium.

As America began to transform itself from a rural to an urban society, the use of liquor and beer began to increase. Along with the rising popularity of alcohol and the opiates came various attempts at suppression. As alcohol flowed into the mainstream of American life—especially in the cities—religious organizations, suffragettes, and other groups involved in urban agitation ranged themselves in violent opposition against the influence of what were considered the devil's two handmaidens. It was not long before the specter of alcohol—which came to the cities at a time when they were undergoing their first gigantic expansion since the Civil War—fell under the sway of Prohibition. Basically a small-town practice, opium and the various elixirs were the first to be proscribed by the Prohibition groups and the zealous reformers.

The end of one era and the beginning of another were demonstrated by the enactment of the Harrison Narcotics Act of 1922, which curbed the use of opium in the form of paregoric in patent medicines.

The Volstead Act, passed in 1919 and repealed in 1933, prohibited the use and manufacture of liquor in the United States. It was America's answer to a problem that posed a direct challenge to its moral foundations. Despite its brief relegation to the national psyche's subconscious during the turbulent expansion westward, the puritanic ethic now began to crystallize in the cities, where it was eagerly taken to the bosom of the churches and other moral urban groups. It would be relevant to examine the history of the Volstead and Harrison acts as precursors of the Marijuana Tax Act, and the way in which they dealt with the problems of alcohol and opium before suppression of marijuana became the main concern of the law.

The Volstead and Harrison acts had their roots in the conflict between the puritanic ethic and its relation to intoxicants. Three norms are intimately connected with this body of values underlying the American ethos. To justify the curbs on intoxicants and narcotics, the first norm applied was that of "control" and its connotation of complete individual responsibility for one's actions. The corollary to this maxim held in disrepute any practice resulting in loss of self-control. The drunkard has relinquished mastery over his physical activities and his judgment is awry. Therefore, according to such reasoning, the substance that led to this condition is evil. The opium users were less clamorous; they tended to fall asleep and were less likely to commit the rash acts of people under the influence of alcohol. Nonetheless, they were also the victim of an outside influence that ruled their faculties because they displayed a physical dependence upon the drug.

The second puritanic ethic applicable to this case dealt with the concept of "undeserved pleasures." It was believed that pleasure was "good" only if it had been earned. The pragmatic bent of the puritanic mind considered sex enjoyable only if it were performed for the sake of procreation. The pleasure motive per se was considered unworthy and debasing to man's nature. This cultural emphasis, although rapidly diminishing in our contemporary society, tends to make Americans feel uneasy and ambivalent about ecstatic experiences of any kind except those that are the by-product or reward of actions considered proper in their own right—such as industry or religious fervor. Those pursuing ecstasy for its own sake are usually condemned for enjoying "illicit pleasure." Thus alcohol and the opiates were scorned because they produced pleasure that the puritanic ethic found reprehensible. Alcohol, however, is more easily condoned by the puritanic mind since the drinker is "punished" for his "illicit pleasure" on the following day—by the hangover.

A self-righteous do-goodism was the third norm to play a role in the suppression of intoxicative substances. Evangelical reformers usually encountered human wrecks who had become totally enslaved to alcohol and opium. They believed that repressive laws were the only way to curb the use of intoxicants for the betterment of the individuals involved as well as of society at large.

Such norms laid the moral groundwork for subsequent legislation. The Eighteenth Amendment and the Volstead Act prohibited the manufacture of alcoholic beverages in the United States and their import, and the Harrison Narcotics Act prohibited the use of opiate drugs for all but medical purposes. Like the Marijuana Tax Act that followed it, the Harrison Act was passed as a revenue measure, slapping exorbitantly high taxes on purveyors of opiate drugs without a license while charging such legitimate licensees as doctors, dentists, veterinarians, and pharmacists a nominal tax. Although justified constitutionally as a revenue measure, the Harrison Act—again like the Marijuana Tax Act—was, in fact, a police measure and was interpreted as such by those enforcing the laws. The result of this flurry of legislative activity was the subsequent establishment of the Federal Bureau of Narcotics in 1930 as an adjunct to the Treasury Department with special jurisdiction over the enforcement of these drug laws.

The same argument advanced for the legislation against alcohol and the opiates were also applied to marijuana. There were some local and state laws against its use at the time, yet generally enforcement was relatively lax. Neither the public nor law-enforcement agencies considered marijuana the problem it has come to be today. Except for the most glaring violations, marijuana use was not deemed important enough to warrant major attempts at enforcement.

The Treasury Department itself considered the problem of minor importance. As late as 1931, its yearly report, "Traffic in Opium and Other Dangerous Drugs," stated:

> A great deal of public interest has been aroused by newspaper articles appearing from time to time on the evils of the abuse of marijuana, or Indian hemp, and more attention has been focused on specific cases reported of the abuse of the drug than would otherwise have been the case. This publicity tends to magnify the extent of the evil and lends color to an inference that there is an alarming spread of the improper use of the drug, whereas the actual increase in such use may not have been inordinately large.

Looking back, it is interesting to note the shift in opinion on the part of the Federal Bureau of Narcotics. When the FBN was agitating for enforcement of anti-marijuana laws and during the Congressional hearings that preceded the passage of the Marijuana Tax Act, the official stand linked the drug with crimes that ranged from rape to murder. In answer to queries at the hearings about whether or not the marijuana addict graduated to heroin or other addictive drugs, the FBN representatives replied in the negative.

A few months later the same point was made before the Senate subcommittee by the FBN in reply to a similar question: "There is an entirely new class of people using marijuana. The opium user is around thirty-five to forty years old. These users are twenty years old and know nothing of heroin or morphine."

When the FBN's Anslinger appeared before a Congressional hearing almost twenty years later, the following exchange took place between him and Senator Price Daniel:

"Now, do I understand from you, that while we are discussing marijuana, the real danger there is that the use of marijuana leads many people eventually to the use of heroin, and causes complete addiction. Is that correct?"

Anslinger agreed: "That is the great problem and our grave concern about the use of marijuana—that eventually, if used over a long period of time, it does lead to heroin addiction."

It would seem, therefore, that the Federal Bureau of Narcotics had drastically revised its outlook on the marijuana question over the past twenty years. Soft-pedaling the link between marijuana and crime, the bureau stressed instead that marijuana's danger lay in the path it beat to heroin addiction.

Pursuing the subject, one of the Senators asked whether "it is or is not a fact that the marijuana user has been responsible for many of our most sadistic, terrible crimes in this nation, sex slayings and matters of that kind?"

This time Mr. Anslinger hedged: "There have been instances of that, Senator. We have had some rather tragic occurrences by users of marijuana. It does not follow that all crime can be traced to marijuana. There have been many brutal crimes traced to marijuana but I could not say that it is a controlling factor in the commission of crimes. . . We are trying to keep away from the marijuana addict, because he is not a true addict. The real problem is the heroin addict."

Dr. Lindesmith comments on this contradiction:

> If it is true that marijuana users were not switching to heroin in 1937, it seems probable that it was the 1937 anti-marijuana law itself that brought about the change. With the risks increased, prices and profits on the now illicit commodity went up, with the result that merchants who had earlier handled one or the other of these drugs, but not both, now began to handle both of them. The marijuana user thus found himself able to purchase heroin from merchants who had previously sold only marijuana.

Following World War II the United Nations assumed responsibility for the international control of drugs. This world-wide forum proved receptive to many of the FBN's views. Hashish was banned in Egypt and opium outlawed in Thailand. Through the adoption of the United Nations Single Convention on Narcotic Drugs in 1961, suppression rather than legalization and punishment rather than humane treatment for addicts became the world-wide norm—just as it was in the United States.

At the direction of the Economic and Social Council of the United States, a commission on narcotic drugs was established. In addition, the Expert Committee on Addiction-Producing Drugs was organized under the World Health Organization (WHO). The organization designated drugs that, for their addictive potential, should be under international control; it also provided other technical information to the commission on Narcotic Drugs. Anslinger, although ostensibly retired since 1962, has been keeping in close touch with these international councils. He emerged in 1967 for an appearance before Senator Fulbright's Foreign Relations Committee where he made a strong plea for the United Nations Single Convention of 1961. This treaty, basically a document reflecting Anslinger's ideas, has become the main instrument toward an international ban on marijuana. The former chief of the Federal Narcotics Bureau remarked on the growing clamor in the United States for liberalization of the marijuana controls. He argued that "if the United States becomes a party to the 1961 Single Convention, we will be able to use our treaty obligations to resist legalized use of marijuana." His words were heeded. On May 25, 1967, the United States became the fifty-seventh country to sign the Single Convention.

Between its adoption by the United Nations in 1961 and the time the United States became a signatory in 1967, the Single Convention was not always without criticism from representatives of the internaional body itself.

In 1965, a member of the Ministry of Health of Brazil asked the commission to show a more humane attitude toward treatment of addicts and a possible reassessment of cannabis. As the United States representative to the commission, Anslinger regarded such questions as particularly unfortunate because they took a view contrary to that of the commission "on the criminogenic action of this narcotic drug."

A recent session of the international body delivered what must be considered a final blow to the spirit of open inquiry as well as internal consistency; it resolved that "the subject should no longer appear on the Commission agenda as the 'question' of cannabis. There should be no question that cannabis presented a danger to society although more and more people were attempting to cast out the necessity of controlling the substance."

The commission's stance was paralleled by the official attitude in the United States. As recently as 1966, Henry L. Giordano, who was Commissioner of Narcotics when the FBN was abolished in 1968, warned members of a Senate subcommittee that "making any broad distinction between the controls and penalties between marijuana and those other narcotics would be a serious mistake."

Answering New York Senator Jacob Javits, he admitted to having no figures on the percentage of crime caused by marijuana users. Instead, he introduced as evidence a document entitled "What Is So Bad About Marijuana," which was nothing more than a rehash of the unverified charges that led to the establishment of the Marijuana Tax Act in 1937. Giordano went on to state that he scorned the "aggressive adolescents at odds with the conventional norms of our society for their use of a drug which has *a worse effect than heroin* and is more intoxicating than alcohol; and the abusive use of which is more likely to lead to insanity . . . and which has been responsible for numerous and varied major crimes."

Again, a long list of vicious crimes were spun out and related to the effects of marijuana: A savage attack on a sixteen-year-old high-school girl who had smoked marijuana prior to the attack; a murder and suicide by a service-station operator in whose pockets were found a package of marijuana cigarettes; and a case of exhibitionism in which the sexual pervert admitted that smoking marijuana had precipitated his indecent exposure to younger girls.

Another case cited as evidence by Giordano concerned a man who, accused of having assaulted a ten-year-old girl, pleaded not guilty on grounds of temporary insanity caused by his smoking of marijuana. Giordano thought this case was a perfect example since it combined all three ingredients—sex, crime, and insanity. The court that tried the man did not quite interpret the marijuana-crime causality chain according to the commissioner's views and the defendant was sentenced to death.

The United States Senate shows a similar resistance to change. In fact, its approach to the marijuana question seems to be exactly at the level of thirty years ago. In a report of the Senate Foreign Relations Committee on the United Nations Single Narcotics Convention, Senator Mike Mansfield noted that there was no opposition to ratification of the treaty to put suppression of marijuana in the category of an international obligation. Continued the Senator: "Mr. President, this convention is supported by the Departments of State, the Treasury Department, and by Mr. H. J. Anslinger, the former Commissioner of the Bureau of Narcotics."

What exactly are the laws that have been so stoutly defended by the enforcement agencies? First of all, the state laws are usually limited to prohibitions of possession or sale of marijuana. But until the May 19, 1969 ruling of the Supreme Court in the case of Dr. Timothy F. Leary, anyone who transferred, acquired, or possessed marijuana was also answerable to the Internal Revenue Department by decree of the 1937 Marijuana Tax Act.

A review of the Leary charges and the defense that precipitated the Supreme Court's decision will serve to clarify the legislation. Dr. Leary was convicted in 1966 under the 1937 Marijuana Tax Act because he had been apprehended entering the United States at Laredo, Texas, with several ounces of marijuana in his automobile for which he had not paid the required $100-per-ounce transfer tax. In so doing, he had simultaneously violated another anti-marijuana law that makes it illegal to import marijuana from abroad without proper authority. He was given a five-to-thirty-year sentence and fined $40,000; and his eighteen-year-old daughter, Susan, who was found with the marijuana, was placed on probation until she reached legal age.

Leary's defense against these two charges has been based on his privilege under the Fifth Amendment to protect himself from self-incrimination. In its ruling, the Supreme Court granted Dr. Leary (and persons in his situation) an absolute defense to prosecution; since all fifty states have laws that make possession of marijuana illegal, to comply with the federal law would expose a person to state prosecution.

The opinion left undisturbed a federal law under which persons who sell marijuana illegally are subject to stiff jail sentences. Moreover, persons can still be convicted under the anti-importation law if it can be shown that they knew the marijuana was not a domestic product. The legality of state laws, of course, is in no way affected.

Since violation of one section of state or federal law is usually accompanied by failure to observe other provisions, sentences can be mounted, one on top of the other. Through the years, sentences of twenty or thirty years have not been uncommon while in one instance a thirty-year-old woman was sentenced to 110 years.

These federal marijuana laws impose the same harsh penalties that are assessed against narcotics offenders. In addition, state penalties, also very severe, rarely distinguish between marijuana and narcotics.

These laws have long been attacked as stable and unyielding by those who have looked at the problem from a more balanced and objective viewpoint. Says Dr. Alfred R. Lindesmith: "The penalty provisions applicable to marijuana users under state and federal laws are about the same as those applied to heroin users. These penalties are entirely disproportionate to the seriousness of the offending behavior and lead to gross injustice and undesirable social consequences. For example, it is well-known that many jazz musicians and other generally inoffensive persons use or have used marijuana. To send these persons to jail is absurd and harmful and serves no conceivable purpose. The moderate or occasional marijuana user is not a significant social menace. Jails and prisons, chronically overcrowded, should be used for those who present a genuine threat to life and property."

Lindesmith raises the question of legislative reform:

> There are more and more indications that the inappropriateness of present United States policy with respect to marijuana is coming to be widely acknowledged, and the need for a genuine legislative examination of this matter is becoming increasingly evident. The 1937 legislation was passed by Congress largely at the behest of the Federal Bureau of Narcotics without any genuine inquiry into the facts. By 1951, marijuana was customarily lumped with other drugs such as heroin, morphine, and cocaine, and the penalties attached to its use were made more severe along with the others. The story was repeated in the 1956 Narcotic Control Act, when the penalties for marijuana violators were again sharply

increased with no more than a casual legislative glance at the actual problem and without even the pretense of an inquiry.

In 1962 the White House Conference on Narcotics and Drug Abuse contained a somewhat cautious recommendation along these lines: "It is the opinion of the panel that the hazards of marijuana per se have been exaggerated and the long criminal sentences imposed on occasional users or possessors are in poor social perspective."

Noting the relatively minor nature of a marijuana offense, the President's Advisory Commission in 1963 suggested the elimination of all mandatory sentences relating to it, while giving judges full discretionary powers in cases of this nature. Despite their ostensible liberal stamp, these recommendations still fail to answer the question as to why there should be a jail sentence in the first place. Lindesmith has this suggestion to offer:

> If it is deemed in the public interest to punish smokers of marijuana, such punishment should ordinarily consist of fines only, up to some maximum of perhaps $500, depending upon the offense and the defendant's ability to pay . . . Police efforts should be focused primarily on the traffic rather than on the user. Persons driving automobiles under the influence of the drug might be fined and deprived of their driving licenses for a period of time. Crimes which could be shown to the satisfaction of a court of law to be linked with the use of marijuana ought to be dealt with about the way that crimes arising from the use of alcohol are handled.
>
> Laws such as this, with penalties of a reasonable nature, would probably be more effective than those now in effect because they would be more enforceable and more in accord with the nature of the problem being dealt with. They would have the effect of reducing the discrepancy that now exists between the laws as written and the laws as they are actually enforced.

The 1967 President's Crime Commission—specifically the Task Force on Narcotics and Drug Abuse—made some strong recommendations for revising the marijuana laws. Individual members suggested that the penalty for possession be reduced to a misdemeanor rather than a felony; Task Force member Dr. M. Rosenthal proposed that criminal sanction against use and possession be entirely removed. The commission's overall recommendations, however, related only to the removal of the mandatory aspects of marijuana penalties and the suggestion that a comprehensive research program be undertaken. An earlier change in the present laws did make federal violators eligible for parole.

Today, the tendency of the news media as well as of public forums is toward more moderate treatment of marijuana. But it is public re-education rather than the collection of additional facts that will determine the modification of the marijuana laws. If one may infer anything from the current attitude of the press, other modifications may well appear within the next few years.

Other factors instrumental in changing the mood of the people are the methods of marijuana law enforcement that run counter to our cherished right of privacy. Quite a number of persons opposed to the legalization of marijuana are even more strongly set against the invasion of a person's home to enforce a law against a personal habit. Many of the "sex" laws still on the books have faltered on exactly these grounds. The informer—another technique commonly used in enforcing the drug laws—is also reprehensible to many persons cherishing democratic ideals.

Furthermore, there are glaring contradictions in the laws themselves. For instance, peyote, mescaline, LSD, and psilocybin have virtually the same psychic effects but the crazy quilt of California laws permits peyote for some Indians, defines mescaline as a narcotic and imposes on its use the same severe penalties as for heroin use, considers LSD a dangerous drug with a misdemeanor charge for possession, while psilocybin is not covered at all. Marijuana—the mildest of hallucinogens, which could not be logically included in the above group—is treated as a narcotic.

Recent adverse publicity has made LSD and other psychedelics illegal in most states. The irony of the marijuana legislation underscores the contradictory nature of the drug laws that have been passed in this country: LSD, the most potent hallucinogen known to man, carries penalties often fifty percent less severe than those for an identical marijuana charge. Despite its slight hallucinogenic action, possession of marijuana on a first offense can carry, in some states, a penalty of up to ten years imprisonment, while LSD possession may not even be illegal. These inconsistencies are ultimately bound to lead to a change in the marijuana laws.

Joseph Lohman, Dean of the University of California (Berkeley) School of Criminology, has pointed out that the marijuana laws, as presently constituted, hold the germ of a host of unnecessary personal tragedies. The new breed of marijuana users—students and other middle-class persons who are not basically antisocial—may be tagged for the remainder of their lives with an arrest record and subsequent social disfavor. This process may at the same time breed a subculture hostile to the law in general. In addition, there is the true criminal element in organized crime that illegal marijuana supports and creates.

Selective enforcement presents another problem. The injustice of the severe penalties for pot violations were never publicly articulated until the white middle class took up the habit; but the minority groups who were the early users of marijuana believed the drug to be relatively harmless while being uncomfortably aware of the disproportionate penalties involved if they were caught indulging the habit. The early biographies of Negro jazz musicians were full of complaints of this nature. That the laws themselves, and especially the enforcement of these laws, are in poor social perspective is emphasized by the facts that the police frequently look the other way when college students are involved, and that the courts often fail to follow the letter of the law, which would otherwise mean inordinately severe sentences.

At the other end of the spectrum, the situation can supply law-enforcement agencies with an excuse to clamp down on types of behavior that are unpopular but not illegal. At best, it results in an unjust distinction between certain lower classes of people who are usually kept under close surveillance by the police, while students and upper socio-economic groups use the drug with impunity.

As these simmering arguments come to a boil, a basic change in the marijuana laws appears imminent, for although the Federal Bureau of Narcotics succeeded in obtaining anti-marijuana legislation, it has not been able to eliminate the drug's popularity. It seems to be always available and, as its use spreads, the old myth and the new reality grow farther and farther apart.

The attempts to suppress marijuana have admittedly failed. The laws against selling and using have never been so severe, arrests have never been so numerous—and the number of users and sellers, never so great. The mushrooming incidence of indulgence among the dominant white middle class pits the law against friends, colleagues, employees, neighbors, and children. The present marijuana situation can be compared to the Victorian sex taboos that still prevailed in the first few decades of the twentieth century. It was not until our major novelists, scientists, and artists made us face our real natures that sex was liberated and entered the mainstream of American life. The same is likely to happen with marijuana.

The shift in views can already be observed in the daily newspapers, as illustrated by two stories that recently appeared in the same week. One, entitled "A Cop Joins a Protest and Career Goes to Pot," featured a young police sergeant in uniform who lighted a marijuana cigarette in the halls of justice before three hundred fellow demonstrators against California's marijuana laws. Narcotics officers prompted arrested Sergeant Richard Bergess and booked him on a charge of possession of marijuana.

Bergess told reporters before being taken into custody that he was "acting in protest and disgust; it was my thing. I did what was right at the time." He declared that his purpose was to show his scorn for a system of laws that allows the free sale of guns while "you can be arrested for the smoking of a harmless vegetable."

The second news story told how Deputy District Attorney Boyd Hornor, of Santa Barbara, California, resigned his office, charging that too much of his time was wasted in prosecuting marijuana users.

"For the first time in the Santa Barbara records," he said, "marijuana complaints exceed either burglaries or auto thefts. The district attorney's office has brought more marijuana felony cases to trial in the local superior court in recent months than virtually all other felony cases combined." He added that "almost every deputy district attorney in Santa Barbara has a marijuana case or two," and he further asserted that "while the law enforcement must be beefed up materially if marijuana is really a threat to society's health and safety, studies show that the drug is not a serious danger and therefore the law should be changed. If marijuana is not the danger it is made out to be, then the district attorney's resources could be better put to use in other fields such as the growing area of consumer fraud."

Interestingly enough, as recent as May, 1968, a bill passed by the New York State Assembly making the sale or distribution of marijuana to minors a crime punishable by a maximum sentence of life imprisonment was sent to Governor Nelson Rockefeller for approval. Only one other state, Ohio, has a statute as tough. Not only did Governor Rockefeller regard the bill as "harsh and regressive," he was immediately pressured from all corners to veto the bill.

The New York Civil Liberties Union complained that this piece of legislation would "make the penalty for selling marijuana cruel and unusual punishment, in violation of the Eighth Amendment to the United States Constitution."

As a result of the telegrams and letters protesting the severity of the bill that flooded the Governor's office, Rockefeller vetoed it. Many legislators who had voted for the bill's passage lamely admitted that they had not understood the full force of the measure until long after its passage. They learned to their surprise that, had their legislation been enacted, a college student giving a single marijuana cigarette to a friend would have been liable to life imprisonment for his act.

The movement to legalize marijuana, both official and unofficial, has been under way for some time. The official movement is called LeMar (the Committee to Legalize Marijuana) and it is not made up of just hippies. On the West Coast, James R. White, a Goldwater conservative and practicing attorney, is the legal counsel for the organization. The marijuana laws, White claims, are "reducing respect for law enforcement, just as prohibition did."

In addition, when the ultraconservative *National Review* recently published Antoni Gollan's lengthy article in favor of legalizing pot, the article stated that at least four prominent conservative writers privately admit smoking pot, and quoted a fifth as saying that the marijuana laws are "unrealistic, repressive and should be repealed or reformulated." Gollan adds that early in 1968 the Young Americans for Reagan, a California-based national conservative organization working to help draft the Governor for President, issued a position paper urging repeal of the marijuana laws.

The paper stated that "if a person is behaving differently from how a moral collectivist wants him to behave and yet is minding his own business, who or what gives the moralist the right to prevent that person's behavior?" This statement concluded that California's tax money would be better spent if police were allowed to devote their energies to solving crimes of violence rather than coercing moral authority. The paper also mentions an astonishing figure of twenty million dollars a year being spent in California alone on detection and imprisonment of marijuana sellers and smokers—with the result that marijuana smoking is more widespread than ever.

Mr. Gollan quotes the United States Constitution in support of his thesis: "Excessive bail shall not be required nor excessive fines imposed or cruel or unusual punishment inflicted." He states that conservatives have generally insisted on a literal reading of the Constitution and its clearly defined restraints upon government from arbitrary or excessive authority. He therefore poses the question as to whether life imprisonment constitutes cruel and unusual punishment for the recreational use of a substance that has been described as having "the abuse potential of a cocktail." He asserts that it has been the feeling of most conservatives that social attitudes and behavior cannot be legislated—in fact, should not be legislated, lest the action do injury to individual liberty and personal prerogative.

Gollan also reports a significant court case challenging the constitutionality of Massachusetts' marijuana laws; the defendants' attorney, Joseph S. Oteri, is also, interestingly enough, counsel for the National Association of Police Officers. In an article titled, "In The Marketplace of Free Ideas: A Look at the Passage of the Marijuana Tax Act," written by Oteri and Harvey A. Silvergate, the authors have this to say:

> Both the Congress and Mr. Anslinger—having long ignored the pleas of medical men and scientists that they take a rational view of the problem—may some day find themselves embarrassed by a court's findings that the entire range of marijuana legislation violates one or more clauses of the United States Constitution. . . .
>
> It would be a sharp blow to the legislative process and to the pride and reputation of legislative bodies if the present laws remain unexamined long enough to force a court to look at the facts and conclude that the marijuana laws were passed without any investigation into what is known by experts—sociologists, psychologists, psychiatrist, pharmacologists, and so forth. This might well happen when the concept of Due Process of Law is interpreted so as to require a legislature to look at the facts before it passes severe penal laws.
>
> Yet the legislatures, including the Congress of the United States,

have thus far chosen to continue accepting the old well-worn myths propagated by men with no scientific objectivity or training.*

Similar cases are in progress in New York and Rhode Island and a bill to remove marijuana from the state narcotics law was recently placed before the Michigan legislature.

Gollan also tells of a Health, Education, and Welfare Department paper circulating in Washington that recommends studying the feasibility of eventually "removing present restrictions on the sale and distribution of marijuana in the same fashion that alcohol is controlled." The liberal *New Republic* also came out for a reappraisal of the marijuana laws. Its March, 1968 issue contained a highly reasoned legal article, asserting that "it is likely that most marijuana arrests in the nation's capital are being made under an unconstitutional law."

And so the marijuana battle continues to rage. The outcome of the test cases now pending in some of the states will be decisive in determining which way the scales of justice will tip.

***Marijuana: Myths and Realities*. Edited by J. L. Simmons, Ph.D., Brandon House © 1967.

CHAPTER NINE

UNDERGROUND POT: THE CRIMINAL ASPECTS

From the Mexican Barrios to the American Suburbs

No matter what the mass media may say, no one syndicate controls the underground market in marijuana. Because of the nature of the drug (it is not physically addictive) and because the plant that produces the drug grows in abundance and is so easily obtainable, it would be a difficult job to monopolize this market. To pin down exactly how pot circulates in the United States, however, is a formidable task.

First of all, most of it is grown in Mexico and makes its way into the United States. There are wholesalers who *are* connected with the Mafia and others who are not; there are middlemen who buy from these wholesalers and are wholesalers themselves; there are street pushers (the retailers) who buy by the pound and sell only $5.00 and $10.00 bags; there are also individual entrepreneurs—campus pushers and hippie pushers—who may purchase the stuff wholesale from Mafia contacts or make the trip to Mexico themselves; and there are the casual users who may come across an opportunity to secure a large amount and then sell it at cost to their friends.

Basically, the way marijuana is wholesaled and retailed in the United States tends to vary with the kind of buyer. The field remains competitive, and anybody who wants to go into the business needs only a small amount of capital. However, for the effort and risk involved, the profits are small.

A market-research analyst, although he would have some trouble obtaining his information, would divide the people who purchase pot in this country into five main groups. Their buying patterns, as with any other product, dictate the ways marijuana is sold.

These five groups are: (1) the urban minority groups (including the ghetto groups—the Negroes, Puerto Ricans and other Spanish-speaking people); (2) the rural minority groups (consisting mainly of poor farm workers, many of them Negroes and Mexican-Americans); (3) the white middle-class students (who are a relatively new market but seem to be outnumbering all the other groups); (4) the hippies (who make use of not only marijuana but also the more potent hallucinogens—peyote, mescaline, LSD, as well as speed); and (5) the group over thirty (artists, intellectuals, writers, and beatniks who went "straight," people who learned to smoke in college or in the service).

All of these groups influence the way marijuana is distributed. According to the law, they are all "criminals" and, because they must take great care in obtaining their supply of marijuana, they all have characteristics in common.

All marijuana, of course, is black market because possession, smoking, sale, and even giving it away are illegal in this country. Most of it comes from Mexico and the Caribbean Islands. It continues to be brought to the United States in shipments ranging from tons to pocketfuls and only a small fraction of the amount is detected by customs officials. Recently the plant has begun to be cultivated domestically by a small percentage of users who have access to out-of-the-way tracts and wish to avoid the difficulty of purchasing the drug underground.

Nobody doubts the central importance of Mexico in growing marijuana for the United States market. Chester Emerick, the Treasury Department's Deputy Commissioner of Customs, declared in 1962 that "ninety-nine percent of our marijuana comes from Mexico," agreeing with a similar statement of the Federal Bureau of Narcotics at about the same time.

Marijuana is cultivated in certain parts of Mexico, where the farmers see an opportunity for greater income than the customary agricultural crops bring. They are usually approached by an American through a middleman who wishes to be assured of a certain supply. They also grow it for their own consumption for although marijuana is illegal in Mexico, smoking it has continued to be a widespread custom and the law is rarely enforced against individual smokers.

The source of supply for the individual Mexican, however, is his own backyard, where he can scatter a handful of seeds that will produce enough marijuana for his own or family use. It is only the large-scale growers who are harassed by the authorities, but some farmers wonder whether it is worth the trouble. They receive approximately fifteen thousand dollars if they grow and harvest a ton of the stuff. Out of that sum they must pay off the local officials, the police, and the local entrepreneurs who make the deals for them—the farmer usually not dealing with the American buyer himself. Rafael Palma, a Mexican police official, described the situation of the marijuana farmer, as an activity undertaken primarily ". . . for the gringoes. It's money Mexico could use and it's a lot more than the farmers could get growing corn and beans. Local residents treat the soldiers like enemies. They refuse to sell them food or supply water. We are just one more plague to these people, like locusts. Just another hardship that must be put up with."

In Mexico the law against marijuana is held in even greater contempt than it is by some groups here in the United States. Since Mexico, however, was a signer of the United Nations Single Narcotic and Drug Act of 1961, they must at least put up a token show of enforcing the laws against mass production of marijuana for export to the United States, even though nothing is done about individual batches growing in backyards.

Enforcement of these laws is far from popular and, as a result, the Bureau of Narcotics subsidizes the Mexican police authorities by supplying them with arms and equipment. The small-town officials, whose first allegiance is to the farmers, seldom give much assistance to the federal Mexican police officials. Thus the source remains a viable one and it is doubtful if it will be eliminated in the near future.

The fortunes reputed to be made from marijuana do not show in the pocketbook of the Mexican farmer growing the hemp plant. Depending on the bulk purchased, it can be bought for as low as $5.00 to $10.00 a pound in Mexico—petty cash to United States entrepreneurs. These prices depend, of course, on the number of hands the product has passed through and the amount purchased. The only customers who seem to pay exorbitant prices for their marijuana are the agents of the Bureau of Narcotics who will, of course, gladly pay any amount as long as they can make an arrest.

One case concerning FBN agents involved a $150,000 payment for a little more than four tons of marijuana, which averages out to approximately $20.00 per pound. In another case a Mexican front man was paid $25.00 a pound by the FBN agents. This would have been an exceptionally good deal on his part if he hadn't been arrested later. Generally, such deals run more along the lines of the one involving Niño Mendoza, who showed up in San Luis Potosi with three-quarters of a ton of marijuana that he had agreed to sell for eleven hundred dollars. This comes to about $7.00 a pound and is a much more realistic price.

Although the Mafia does not control the marijuana traffic, there is no denying that various Mafia groups and other gangster organizations are involved in the distribution. Marijuana, as such, is not a highly profitable business proposition like heroin, the backbone of the Mafia establishment. But it is profitable enough, as is evident from the following statement quoted by Dr. Walton in his book, *Marijuana: America's New Drug Problem*. He tells of an interview with a drug dealer during one of the investigations in the thirties, before the passage of the federal legislation:

> The gangster remarked: "Marijuana is the coming thing."
>
> "But," I protested in surprise, "marijuana is not a habit-forming drug like morphine or heroin; and besides, it's too cheap to bother with."
>
> He laughed. "You don't understand. Laws are being passed now by various states against it, and soon Uncle Sam will put a ban on it. The price will then go up, and that will make it profitable for us to handle."

Chief among the reasons why the supply cannot be monopolized and continues to come from a combination of entrepreneurs is that marijuana is a plant that, after drying, needs no other preparation (unlike heroin, which involves a complicated process of chemical manipulations including the hiring of chemists, laboratories, and the like). Also, unlike heroin, which is controlled by huge investment from the top of the Mafia establishment, marijuana can be obtained in almost any amount, from ounces to tons, direct from the producer in Mexico.

Reports from the Federal Bureau of Narcotics show that each

urban area is serviced by a variety of suppliers, with the marijuana originating from different Mexican localities. Inclusive of an initial investment for the payment and transportation, an amount of 100 pounds can be purchased for approximately $15.00 to $25.00 per pound and smuggled into any American border city, whence it finds its way to other parts of the United States to be sold for $100 to $300 per pound.

Purchases of more than 500 pounds usually lower the price to as little as $10.00 a pound, and when the total purchase reaches into the tons, the rock-bottom price of $5.00 to $7.00 per pound is normal. It is obvious, then, that there is money to be made from marijuana dealing. As a result, organized crime is handling a good deal of the traffic. The public impression, however, that the amount of money involved in the dealings is astronomical is false. This is mainly due to the quotes publicized by the Federal Bureau of Narcotics that generally exaggerate the commercial values of drug seized.

A news headline reading "MILLION DOLLARS IN POT SEIZED AND DOPE RING ARRESTED" usually originates from the press-release machine of government agencies involved in the seizures (the Federal Bureau of Narcotics and the United States Customs). They give the "retail" figures placing the worth at approximately $1.00 a cigarette. This is the highest possible value that can be placed on marijuana, for it is rarely sold for that amount even when pieced out in single cigarettes.

For example, if the United States Customs seize a ton of marijuana (2,000 pounds) it is more than likely that it was paid for at the rate of $7.50 per pound, which would make the wholesale value $15,000. If the Customs office impounded it at this stage of the game, the price for it would most realistically be the wholesale price. Later it will be broken down into kilos (2.2 pounds) or pounds that sell for $100 to $300, depending upon the area of the country and the distance from the Mexican border. Afterward, it will be broken down into ounces that sell for up to $35.00 then divided into nickel bags (1/5 of an ounce and called nickel bags because each sells for $5.00—according to a junkie terminology that equates a dollar with a penny). This nickel bag is good for approximately 15 to 20 thin marijuana cigarettes. Only on very rare occasions are these cigarettes further retailed for the price of $1.00 each.

Following their own outlandish reasoning the authorities, by estimating that a ton yields 3,000,000 cigarettes, figure that the original ton purchased for $15,000 is worth $3,000,000. This would be like putting the price tag of a Fifth Avenue evening gown on a batch of silkworm cocoons.

The newspapers are replete with this type of reasoning—the most recent being an incredibly exaggerated estimate in which the original $7.50 per pound paid for marijuana in Mexico was inflated to $7,200 per pound when New York State Police and FBN agents seized a mere 7 pounds of pot and tagged the booty at $50,000.

Thus it can be seen that from the pot entrepreneur's point of view, big money can only be made if the original purchasers sold the individual marijuana cigarettes at the retail level themselves. This is never done, however, since anyone who has the required investment to purchase a large amount (say, a ton for $15,000) is not very likely to be caught selling individually rolled cigarettes for 50 cents each on the streets of New York. The profits are dispersed among a large number of middlemen who break up the marijuana bulk along the way before it reaches the streets.

If it is purchased in large amounts, as is usually the case with the wholesale organizations, the ton is usually broken up into 20-to-100-pound lots and sold to middlemen for $75.00 to $150 per pound. The same 20-to-100-pound lots purchased in Mexico (with the required smuggling across the American border to follow) would sell for a maximum of $50.00. As already noted, in the United States a pound is usually sold by the middleman to the street-level distributor for anywhere between $100 to $300. The user and smaller street pusher sometimes buy in ounces for which they pay $20.00 to $35.00 an ounce and the actual user will purchase the nickel bags (1/5 of an ounce) for $5.00. There are, of course, dozens of variations to the above breakdown in "packaging," including the "B" or box, the "dime bags" (a $10.00 bag usually 2/5 or 1/2 ounce), and so on.

Not all marijuana, as has been indicated, comes from the larger gangster organizations. Pot circulates more freely than is generally realized. A good proportion is smuggled into the United States across the Mexican border in the pockets of college students, in the trunks and hollow side panels of automobiles, and even through the mails. However, importing in quantities of more than five hundred pounds to take advantage of the lowest possible price requires considerable investment capital, direct contacts with either the Mexican farmer himself or a front man, a willingness to accept the many risks involved—including arrest—a means of smuggling the marijuana into this country, and an existing organization to oversee the whole operation. The established Mafia organizations are cognizant of the risks involved and do not want to jeopardize their organizations for minimal profits in activities that are likely to bring trouble. The much higher profits involved in the heroin racket are, therefore, usually preferred by these syndicates.

The La Guardia Report of the 1940's, examining this question, negated the concept of a large single group in control of the marijuana traffic; instead, it concluded that it was most likely a combination of smaller entrepreneurs—a still-valid conclusion.

After everything has been arranged in Mexico and the purchase made, the next step for the more sizeable operation is to smuggle the marijuana across the border into the United States. This involves a half-ton, or five hundred pounds at the very least, and has nothing to do with the small-time dealers, such as tourists, students, and professors who return from Mexico bringing back the relatively small amounts—usually five pounds or so—they need to keep themselves supplied for approximately a year.

An example of the large operator was the case of Victor Bono. Despite the myths propagated by the popular press, his was not a vast operation involving hundreds of people, but merely a group of six cohorts. Operating on the West Coast, he imported bulk lots running to approximately one ton; at one point a raid on Bono's house yielded one hundred pounds of marijuana and a small arsenal of weapons.

When the police began to crack down on Bono's enterprise, they apprehended one member of his gang with a truck containing three thousand pounds of marijuana. The subsequent arrest of other members of the Bono group resulted in the confiscation of nine hundred more pounds of marijuana—which was in the process of being smuggled across the border when the guards stopped them. In a period of approximately two months ten thousand pounds of marijuana were seized. Apart from the Bono ring, however, very few operations of this size exist.

More common are the small-time lawbreakers who, aware of the marijuana market, try to make a killing, or petty gangsters who see a chance for an independent business operation. In this class we find the weekend flyer who smuggled approximately one to three hundred pounds in his Piper Cub each weekend from Mexico; the motel owner in southern California who would drive down to Mexico approximately once a month and return with four hundred to five hundred pounds in various panels of his car; the California auto mechanic who had welded special compartments to the underside of his truck for smuggling marijuana; and the Texas aviation worker who would drive down occasionally and return with his spare tire full of marijuana.

All this activity, independent and otherwise, has actually led to a decline in the price of pot during the last few years in the United States. Competition—the American way—has operated to the prime advantage of the marijuana smoker.

Once the marijuana arrives in the United States, it is distributed through dealers (called at various levels "pushers," "connections," "score boys," "newsies," and so on). Underground distribution by these dealers involves a gallery of characters—the street-corner punk employed by the gangster element, Puerto Ricans, Negroes, and Mexican-Americans who sell to their own minority groups, and hippies and students who sell to members of their groups.

In the southwestern United States the Mexican-American smokers who do not grow their own in their backyards buy it from Mexicans or Mexican-Americans who deal in marijuana and cross back and forth between points on both sides of the border.

Not surprisingly, the anti-marijuana laws in the Border States are the most severe in the country. The West Coast areas rely principally on enterprising Californians who do their own importing. It is the northern urban areas with their vast ghettoes that continue to support the syndicate-type operation still extant. The upper-level distribution apparatus that imports marijuana in bulk is the source of the weed for distributors to this minority-group market—consisting mainly of Negroes and Puerto Ricans.

Distribution above street-level pushing is very complex, as in any large enterprise. Once the marijuana is in this country, word of its availability goes out to the customary contacts. The dealer, who usually buys from the importer at this stage, purchases an amount ranging from twenty to one hundred pounds. The prices vary depending on the distance from the Mexican border and the drug's scarcity in the locality. Once the dealer has purchased his supply, he will contact the street pusher who buys in smaller lots—usually pounds. Although the market is changing rapidly because of the influx of the middle-class user, it is still a good estimate to say that half of the marijuana imported into the United States is sold by the street-level pusher who works at it regularly, building up a clientele of regular smokers.

The street pusher will net approximately one hundred to three hundred dollars per week, depending on the volume of business. Although he may not know who his importer is, he may know one or two middlemen who buy from the importer and sell to the street pusher. He must know several such dealers to maintain a source of supply in case one dealer is out of stock. Compared with the selling of heroin—which is usually looked down upon in the community—pushing marijuana carries no stigma in the urban ghettoes. This is especially true in the Puerto Rican neighborhoods of New York City. Smoking pot is a commonplace on the Caribbean Islands; it is carried over as a custom to New York City.

Although circumspection is the word and sales are made only to those inspiring trust—mainly members of their own minority group—and involvement with hard drugs such as morphine and heroin is avoided, there are still occasional arrests. For this reason the street pusher tends to be in his mid-twenties, and if he can stay "clean" for a period of time, his profits are usually invested in some legitimate business, with marijuana relegated to personal use from then on. Some crossover of market territories does occur as, for example, when the street pusher sometimes sells to the campus pusher unable to make contact with a higher-level dealer.

The street pusher's profits are not particularly high. Purchase of a few pounds for which he will pay approximately $100 or more in New York City ($50.00 to $75.00 on the West Coast) may yield him several times his investment capital. However, it involves an arduous cleaning and packaging process of the marijuana tobacco. Afterward, he must go out and find his clientele. This involves delivering the marijuana tobacco to various bars, coffeehouses, and special hangouts. A host of discreet separate transactions often requires more time than the profits warrant.

Disposing of a pound may involve seeing as many as sixty

people, with most of these plumping for no more than $5.00 and $10.00. The ritual that the street pusher must observe as part of the social custom of selling marijuana means turning on with his purchasers, thus producing a subsequent loss of time and money. Further losses are suffered in credit dealings—often necessary if he is to maintain the steady clientele he needs—and delinquent payers are another risk of the trade.

One final problem that constantly confronts the street pusher in the city is the possibility, however remote, of arrest; he therefore tries to keep enough capital on hand for bail, lawyers, and the impounding of his car, if it is found to contain marijuana.

The street pusher in the urban ghetto may start out with high hopes of big profits for little work, but disillusion soon sets in. The ghetto types attracted to this means of livelihood usually dislike working regularly for others at routine tasks for low wages. At first, most of them enjoy turning on friends and usually "dig" their "work." It is not long, however, before they realize that pushing marijuana for profit is not the quickest way to riches. Many an experienced street pusher, if he wishes to remain in the business, becomes a higher-level dealer or importer himself, or drops out of the business completely. The more hardened move on to other drugs, such as heroin.

One of the best accounts of marijuana distribution in the urban ghetto was presented in the La Guardia Report and it is still applicable today. The investigators found at the time two main channels for the distribution of marijuana cigarettes—the independent street peddler and the tea pad. Today the tea pad has mainly disappeared.

The La Guardia Report investigators encountered particular difficulties in analyzing the street pusher's methods because of the reason mentioned earlier—his tendency to sell only to those persons he knows to be of small risk potential. After some months of ingratiating themselves with people in ghetto neighborhoods, the investigators found that they could purchase marijuana in various grills, restaurants, and other hangouts when they made contact with someone who could introduce them to a street peddler making the regular rounds of these places. They also found on rare occasions that public guides and terminal porters would help them to establish contact between purchaser and street peddler. At the time, of course, the ban on marijuana was not as stringently enforced as it is today and public marijuana smoking, such as occurred in lavatories of dance halls, is less evident now than it was then.

The report revealed specific sections in the city of New York where the sale of marijuana appeared to be localized—the Harlem district and the Broadway area running from 42nd Street to 59th Street. Today such sections include Greenwich Village; the East Village; the lower East Side, especially the area around the Seward Park houses; the upper West Side area along Broadway and north of the Lincoln Center; the Broadway-Amsterdam area of the West Side from 86th Street to 96th Street; and the 3rd Avenue-Washington Street area near Tremont Avenue in the Bronx.

The urban street pusher has not changed much over the years since the La Guardia Report was first issued. With the influence of the new market of the young, white middle class, however, many of the former street pushers have now become dealers supplying the campus and hippie pushers, who are the equivalent of ghetto street pushers in their own environment.

The system of marijuana traffic on campus is a bit more erratic than that of the street-level pusher. The campus distributor usually chooses to push marijuana because he is involved in the pot-smoking scene on campus and sees an opportunity to make a few extra dollars. If he has developed a few connections for securing pot, he buys a larger amount and sells some to his pot-smoking friends, and becomes a "pot pusher" for a short period of his college career.

Since he has most likely been smoking pot for some time, he has no moral qualms about his occupation—particularly if he is acquainted with the true facts about the drug. He invariably has quite a few close friends who periodically seek to buy a small amount of grass and, after awhile, he becomes the source for the marijuana.

Although pot is becoming easier to obtain, most students do not exactly relish the idea of having to go into town and hang around some seedy neighborhood waiting for their connection. Knowing someone on campus makes the procedure a lot easier. Rather than spend an hour or a day waiting around to obtain a supply, it is far more convenient to obtain marijuana from someone close by—invariably a student himself. The campus connection, therefore, is commonly the result of "natural selection"—he is the one most adept at copping grass and subsequently gravitates to becoming a pusher as he begins buying for his friends.

Because the campus types are more imaginative and far more mobile than their counterparts in the ghetto, their source is not always restricted to the street-level dealer. As a matter of fact, many a campus pusher started his career after returning from Mexico with a generous quantity of the weed in his suitcase. Since he obtains his supply not only from the higher-level dealer but may also be his own complete organization (that is, he makes the contact in Mexico, smuggles the supply across the border himself and sells it himself), he eliminates the group of middlemen who take a cut of the profits as marijuana is distributed. Campus dealers may also have friends overseas or in Mexico who will gladly mail them some of the commodity.

It is from these students overseas that a new trend in the pot scene has been initiated—hashish use—on American college campuses. It is approximately five to ten times more potent than simple marijuana tobacco. Since it comes in concentrated form, it is far easier to smuggle into the country. Because of the many students traveling abroad—to Europe, North Africa, India, the Far East—it is prevalent chiefly among those of the upper-income groups. Hashish is usually smoked Western style in America; that is, it is either ground to a fine powder and mixed with regular cigarette tobacco and smoked as a reefer; mixed with regular marijuana to make it more potent; or smoked in the long, thin-stemmed bamboo opium pipe.

Thus we see that the campus pusher has established himself as a far more versatile entrepreneur than his ghetto cousin. He can easily jump on a plane (at half-rate student fares), wing down to Mexico and pick up a batch of the weed; or vacation in Europe or India and return with enough hashish to pay his student fees for the college term.

Also, up to the last few years the student pusher was relatively free from the danger of being detected and arrested. The campus was a sacrosanct area and, because of the clannishness of students, he would usually come in contact only with those people he knew and trusted. Knowledge of marijuana smoking rarely transgressed the clique of pot-smoking students.

In the last few years, however, undercover agents, posing as students and hippies, have infiltrated many of the nation's campus groups and a number of arrests have been made. Because this has made the "career" more precarious than it once was, the campus pusher usually practices his trade for only part of his college career and thereby shortens the risk. A recent article in *Esquire* Magazine* tells the story of a campus pusher:

> I pushed in my senior year at the University of Michigan, starting, I remember, after I quit this incredibly boring job showing early-morning educational movies. We were sick of buying lousy grass at exorbitant prices around Ann Arbor, so over Thanksgiving we all chipped in and bought a pound in New York through one of our business associates who lived there and knew a fairly reliable contact. It cost four of us about thirty-five dollars apiece and after weighing it on these great home-made blind-justice-type scales we each wound up with four honest ounces.
>
> Then the idea hit—we could sell a couple, make back our investment, and still have buckets to smoke ourselves. So, we cut the stuff up—this is a technique we eventually got down to a real science—and packaged the ounces in baggies. Now we had to find a market.
>
> At the time, see, we were just looking for a few friends who might want a decent deal, and we'd come out with free grass. So I phoned up a chick I knew who smoked quite a bit and asked her to look around. About a half-hour later she called back with an order for three ounces. We were in business. Our pound went within two days and people were lined up begging for more. What could we do?
>
> You have to understand that this is a pretty common way for pushers to get started. They're not these crummy, slinky, little junkies you read about turning school kids on to pot and dirty pictures. It's the puritan ethic, people, the capitalist way—make a buck. Sure, simple supply and demand—like loan companies and bootleg liquor—hell, like used-car lots and Gimbel's basement. Nobody's a nonprofit organization. One of my partners is an economics major. He filled us in on the real story: just business as usual in the true American tradition.
>
> Before I started pushing I was a long-haired sometime-student Ann Arbor fringe member, cashing my monthly check from upper-suburbia home, and after I started I was just the same—only I was independently wealthy, my parents could save their money for Miami Beach. I mean I didn't make a fortune—just enough

*Reprinted by permission of *Esquire* Magazine © 1967 by Esquire, Inc.

for records and repairs on my car and of course reinvestment.

After our first success we decided the market could easily bear a kilo at a time—which is two-point-two pounds (thirty-five ounces) and costs usually around two hundred and fifty dollars—naturally the more you buy the cheaper it is.

After a few false starts it was decided that purchasing kilos (2.2 pounds) would give the best payoff for the money they had to invest. Their sources were mainly higher-level dealers in Detroit and New York. During their short career in pot pushing they never did purchase marijuana from Mexico. The article describes one of the trips to Detroit to cop some grass:

We alternated buying between Detroit and New York, and although New York City was more chancy, because of the distance, the grass was infinitely better and a lot closer to the real weight—never more than an ounce or two off. Detroit was dishonest through and through. One time sticks in my mind. The contact—he'd gotten over his flu, I guess—called us later in March with a great deal of good grass. And he was anxious to get rid of it. All three of us drove in the next afternoon bulging with money and went up to his crummy room. He had a friend along, a dark greasy guy with his two-year-old daughter, who cried the whole goddam time. There's a technique to buying; first you bullshit, sit around and talk about business, busts, play the guitar, look at his psychedelic pictures. Everybody's real friendly and phony. Nervous.

Then you say, "Well, we'd like a kilo."

They go, "Yeah, sure, fine"—give you some wine. You wander around a little bit more and finally you ask what's the price. You look at their eyes which start to sneak all over the place.

"Two ninety," they say.

"What? Two ninety! Come on, we never pay more than two and a half. That's the standard rate."

And you hassle. . . .

The campus pushers also showed more flair in merchandising their ware than the ghetto connections. First of all, their method of packaging was far more interesting than the usual nickel bag purchased on a street corner. Marijuana comes in a loose pile of roots, stems, and leaves or is sometimes compressed into different-sized blocks. A pound is cut up, cleaned, and packaged for resale. Chopping it up in a grater and straining it until it is fine ensures a better product. Seeds are mashed and sometimes mixed in. Top-grade pot usually has all these seeds and stems removed and contains just the finely ground leaves. These campus pushers decided that this laborious procedure would cut sharply into their profits.

"The trick is not to cut the stuff too fine because the customer would much rather buy a fuller bag of crap than a thinner bag of really beautiful stuff."

They measured the ounces by eye—a pound was divided into approximately sixteen equal piles, then packed in plastic "baggies." If they had been cheated in the purchase of their pound from the dealer, the campus pusher would pass the shortage along to his own customers; if they did receive a full pound, then each customer would get a full ounce. In one instance where the marijuana had been cured in sugar (a quick way of drying it) that eventually shrank it up to almost nothing, the contents were beefed up with green tea to make it look as if there were more marijuana. Other adulterants used to flesh out some meager marijuana buys were catnip (which looks, burns, and smells like marijuana) and some kinds of pipe tobacco.

The campus entrepreneurs figured on a three-hundred-percent return on their investment. An ounce was sold for twenty-five dollars (for which they paid approximately eight dollars); five dollars worth, which should be one-fifth of an ounce, involved even greater chicanery because they would divide an ounce into seven bags instead of the usual five.

The dropouts of society, the real hippies, smoke pot regularly if they do use marijuana. Although they like the experience and the altered perception produced by this mild hallucinogenic weed, the mainstay of their subculture is acid—LSD. Most hippie dealers, like the student pushers, obtain their own marijuana either from Mexico or street-level contacts. Hippie entrepreneurs traveling back and forth across the Mexican-American border bring back with them adequate supplies.

In this group is also found the largest percentage of those who "grown their own." Having the time and the patience to cultivate their own crop, they grow the weed in window flowerpots, on rooftops, in backyards, in rooms, lofts, basements under artificial lighting, and wherever else they can find suitable planting ground. The street-level dealers who supply the urban ghettoes are not popular sources among the hippies.

Hippie communities, which are under greater pressure from the authorities, tend to stock up on larger quantities than is usual among students and the minority groups in order to lessen the risk of being caught with the drug and because generally they consume more of the weed. Because the hippie pushers usually tend to be younger and less mature than campus or ghetto counterparts (and like the ghetto pusher, more closely watched by the police) they suffer a higher percentage of arrests than the campus pusher.

Another differentiating factor of this group is that some hippie pot sellers are only peripherally interested in profits and often obtain the drug for their own peer group after a collection has been made. In other words, the distributor at this hippie subculture level is not profit-oriented but rather like the person who, after a collection has been made, runs down to the corner grocery for a few six-packs of beer; he is not interested in dividing and packaging his products for profit.

Their over-thirty elders who smoke marijuana cut a wide swathe in society. They're usually settled in their habits and life style and do not smoke as frequently as their younger counterparts. They may have started smoking as students, in the military, during the Beatnik period, or were turned on by bohemian friends. This group includes, among others, musicians, artists, writers, and professors.

Leading a more stable life than the smokers in the ghettoes, the students, or the hippies, they have a more difficult time obtaining marijuana and therefore do not smoke as often. Very few of these people are pushers themselves unless members of their peer group turn on quite often.

Other individuals with fairly well regulated lives who reside in the suburbs and are employed in various respectable businesses and professions, frequently obtain their supplies from people they have smoked with in their youth and with whom they have kept in contact for this purpose. Should they have the opportunity to be in Mexico they might also import a few kilos upon return. For as little as fifty dollars they can keep themselves in supply for the year.

Because the over-thirty smoker has more to lose and has developed more respect for society, he is usually the most cautious type of smoker. Yet there is almost no risk at all for this group of smokers, if they choose their sources carefully—for who would suspect marijuana smoking in the suburbs?

CHAPTER TEN

POT AND THE GI: THE MILITARY SCENE

The Grass from Panama to Vietnam

In the military environment, where young men from every level of society are thrown together to work as an efficient force, the arbitrary standards of society often become of lesser import. Especially in the chaos of wartime, social taboos become meaningless and social infractions, unless extremely serious, are usually overlooked.

The military code, although it may seem rather strict in certain areas, has not willingly adopted many of the civilian cultural taboos. It has always had a more-or-less realistic outlook in such matters as drinking, wenching, and hell-raising. Aware that the young soldier must let off steam if he is to remain an efficient part of the military structure, the brass has always made allowances for extracurricular activities frowned upon in civilian life.

As far as marijuana smoking is concerned, the military knows that the habit is picked up through contact with other young men in uniform who turn on regularly. The grab bag of social backgrounds found in the military environment allows the soldiers an insight into a whole spectrum of novel experiences, making this one of the basic learning processes in the life of a youth who may never have drunk anything more potent than soda pop.

Back in 1925 the young American soldiers protecting the Panama Canal Zone were not much different from those scattered throughout the world today. It was a known fact that the men stationed in the Canal Zone had been smoking marijuana for some time, having picked up the habit from the local Panamanians. The military was aware of the practice, but they regarded it as a harmless diversion. However, the late twenties saw the emergence of the "Marijuana Menace" scare, and accordingly, pressure was placed upon the military to examine the drug's use in Panama.

This resulted in the first real marijuana study under American auspices, an investigation conducted in the Panama Canal Zone by the United States Army in 1925. A committee was appointed to study the extent of use and the effects of the drug, and to recommend steps that might be taken to prevent the practice—if it was found to be harmful.

The Army's committee consisted of the Chief Health Officer of the Panama Canal Department of Civil Affairs; the Chief of the Division of Police and Fire; the Department Judge Advocate; the Chief of the Board of Health Laboratories; the Superintendent of the Corazal Hospital for the Insane; and a representative of the United States Navy's Medical Corps acting in an advisory capacity. The committee, called the Panama Canal Zone's Governor's Committee, conducted its investigation from April to December, 1925, and reached the following conclusions: "There is no evidence that marijuana as grown here is a habit-forming drug in the sense in which the term is applied to alcohol, opium, cocaine, etc., or that it has any appreciably deleterious influence on the individual using it."

By 1931, with the anti-marijuana groups gaining prominence, a second Canal Zone study was conducted by the U.S. Army Medical Corps, this time assisted by the offices of the Fifteenth Naval District. This study was far more ambitious than the first and was performed by hospitalizing thirty-four soldiers who had admitted to smoking marijuana. For the period of the study they were permitted to use marijuana freely (the variety used was grown in the Canal Zone Experimental Gardens to assure uniformity of product).

To determine whether the drug was habit-forming, the researchers would periodically withdraw the marijuana supply and observe the subjects for withdrawal symptoms. Each individual soldier was given a complete neuropsychiatric examination and a clinical study before and after smoking marijuana. Further effects were checked by an additional and extensive clinical study following the withdrawal of the drug.

The results of the second study were published in the *Military Surgeon,* the journal of the Association of Military Surgeons of the United States (Nov., 1933, p. 274). The conclusions reached were much the same as those that had been arrived at eight years earlier: "Marijuana as grown and used on the Isthmus of Panama is a mild stimulant and intoxicant. It is not a 'habit-forming' drug in the sense that the derivatives of opium, cocaine, and such drugs are, as there are no symptoms of deprivation following its withdrawal."

The study also analyzed the record of known marijuana smokers to see if the drug was the cause of crime or antisocial behavior. The investigations found that: "Delinquencies due to marijuana smoking which result in trial by military court are negligible in number when compared with delinquencies resulting from the use of alcoholic drinks, which also may be classed as a stimulant and intoxicant." The report went on to say that marijuana presented no threat to military discipline and "that no recommendations to prevent the sale or use of marijuana are deemed advisable."

Nevertheless, these two reports created quite an uproar. Newspapers and magazines attacked them viciously for they saw one of their most lurid topics of reportage snatched away from them.

The editor of the *Military Surgeon,* United States Army Col. James M. Phelan, commented on the attacks in an article entitled "The Marihuana Bugaboo." He stressed the triviality of the effects of marijuana use: "The smoking of the leaves, flowers and seeds of *Cannabis sativa* is no more harmful than the smoking of tobacco or mullen or sumac leaves. The legislation in relation to marijuana is ill-advised. It branded as a menace and a crime a matter of trivial importance. It is hoped that no witch hunt will be instituted in the military service over a problem that does not exist."

Thus ended the first confrontation between pot and the military—all in all, a reasonable outcome.

During World War II and the Korean War large-scale marijuana use was reported among the troops. Again the military overlooked the practice as a trivial occurrence. It was overshadowed by the real problem of addiction to opium, especially among the soldiers in the Far East.

In late 1967, stories of American GI's smoking pot on the Vietnam battlefield suddenly hit the newspapers. Allowing the soldier to take his fling as he finds it has always been an unspoken tradition with the military, but widely reported usage of pot in Vietnam was deemed a blot on the escutcheon of the American fighting force stationed there.

John Steinbeck IV, son of the Nobel Prize-winning novelist, added to the fire of aroused public opinion by stating, upon his return from a year's duty in Vietnam that three-fourths of the GI's there smoke marijuana.

The Army Public Information machine reacted with alacrity to assuage the uproar created by the reports. Brig. Gen. Winant Sidle, the Saigon information chief at United States headquarters at the time, made light of young Steinbeck's allegations despite the fact that in 1967 more United States servicemen in Vietnam were arrested for smoking marijuana than for any other major single offense.

In an Associated Press report, the Army's then Provost Marshal, Brig. Gen. Harley Moore, Jr., admitted that several thousand out of almost half-a-million GI's might be turning on. Brushing aside the earlier Army reports and the expressed medical opinion to the contrary, he indicated his belief that lighting up a joint led to irrational behavior and violence, more so than would the indulgence of alcohol. His biggest concern, though, was his conviction that the brain soaked in pot fumes would be dulled and unable to function in battle.

Newsmen, interviewing GI's after the story broke, found that many a pointman or rifleman on patrol in enemy territory turns on not because he's looking for a different kind of kick, but simply to overcome a basic human and particularly martial emotion: fear. The boredom of war coupled with fighting an elusive enemy make the conflict in Vietnam one where the guard at the gate, the sentinel at the barbed-wire perimeter, and the radio operator monitoring suspicious sounds play key roles in the conduct of the war. Lighting up a joint doesn't make time go faster but it does make a task of drudgery easier to bear, according to many GI's.

The latest study, conducted by Army psychiatrist Captain Wilfred Postell, the results of which were published in 1969 in the official *Vietnam Medical Bulletin* under the heading "Marijuana Use in Vietnam: A Preliminary Report" found that thirty-five percent of the troops turned on.

One of the biggest scandals to emerge out of the Army's marijuana investigations was the discovery that the same GI's confined for pot offenses to the Long Binh stockade, twenty-five miles north of Saigon, were blissfully whiling away their sentences with a supply of grass. How the contraband substance entered the stockade gates is a matter of conjecture. Despite a massive ring of security, an inordinate amount of military goods still manages to get stolen and the Viet Cong learn of classified secrets. Pot, like water, finds its level even in tightly guarded premises. Undoubtedly, it was smuggled in, either through Vietnamese civilians employed in the camp or by way of the guards.

Marijuana, if not growing profusely in Vietnam as it does in such neighboring countries as Laos, Burma, Northern Thailand, and Cambodia, is still readily available there. Located as it is between the world's notorious opium-producing areas, Vietnam has for centuries been a way station for all manner of drugs. Prior to the war, tons of opium and marijuana passed through its ports to destinations all over the world.

A whole new breed of Vietnamese batmen have sprung up from the war's dragon seeds. They are to be found wherever there is a congregation of American GI's. A few words of pidgin English and piasters (Vietnam's monetary unit) smooth the way to fulfillment of whatever the soldier's wish may be. In such Rest & Recreation centers as Vung Tau on the South China Sea coast, the serviceman only has to turn to the nearest street urchin to cop a supply that may last him his year's tour of duty.

In Bien Hoa, the giant military complex just outside Saigon, the connection can be made in any one of hundreds of establishments catering to GI needs—bars, laundries, car washes, souvenir stands. Americans stationed or spending leave in Saigon go to Soul City, a few seedy waterfront blocks. A discreet raising of the fingers over the bar to indicate the number of joints desired is all mama-san needs to know to fill the request. Most brothels stock marijuana as do the individual girls, who sell it as a profitable sideline.

The Indian hemp plant is most widespread in Chau Doc Province near the Cambodian border in the Mekong Delta. According to GI's in the know, the "Cambodian Red," as it is called, is prime-quality stuff—superior to anything that can be obtained in the States. A pack of twenty joints, usually prerolled in American filter cigarettes emptied of their previous contents and filled with marijuana, sells for the piaster equivalent of one dollar.

Individual joints sell for about twenty to thirty piasters apiece (ten to fifteen cents). GI experts can tell which pack out of the numerous brand names carried by a street vendor contains marijuana cigarettes. They recognize it by the way the cellophane has been sealed on a regular pack of American cigarettes.

Marijuana's relative cheapness in Vietnam is perhaps one reason why GI's there turn on with greater frequency than they might in the States. The Vietnamese pot, besides, is a good deal more potent. Although the variety acquired in the Highlands, home of the Montagnard tribes, is somewhat roughly cut, the quality in other parts of the country is of an extremely fine grade. With the chopping mainly done by women, the finished product is usually the pothead's dream of a smooth joint.

A good deal of the marijuana sold in Vietnam comes from Laos and Cambodia. Vietnamese in these border regions carry on a lively trade with their neighbors and a sizeable share of illegally acquired products, such as United States Aid materials and merchandise stolen from the Saigon docks, is exchanged for marijuana, which is carried to the American centers hidden in baskets filled with market product.

The United States military establishment is convinced that the Viet Cong control the trade as a means of demoralizing American troops. A notice widely posted on Army boards across South Vietnam in 1967 said that "the enemy is the big pusher." It went on to note that "the use of marijuana in Vietnam not only endangers the life of the user but also the lives of those depending upon him for the successful accomplishment of his mission. The VC are much aware of the effects of the drug and are instrumental in providing a supply." It urged soldiers to report any suspicion of its use by Army personnel, warning that the "effects of this drug, while not necessarily fatal, are serious."

Although it is doubtful that they are the actual masterminds behind the traffic in marijuana, there is every reason to believe that the Viet Cong stand only to gain from it. Most of the illegal trade takes place in areas where the Communists exert an overt or covert control, taxing all goods that pass through their territory. The Viet Cong also maintain a strong grip on the numerous bars and establishments catering to Americans, the proceeds of which they use to supplement their accounts receivable. A more likely possibility, silently held by Criminal Investigation Division agents, is that of Vietnamese government officials sticking a well-glued finger in the drug traffic and protecting it from outside harassment.

The CID agents in Vietnam, whose initial concern there was mainly with black-market operations and currency violations, have now shifted a major part of their attention to curbing the drug traffic. Often posing as GI's, they busted some seven hundred soldiers in 1967 compared to 238 the previous year. Given the military build-up that took place in 1967, their success cannot be considered spectacular. Much of this stems from the caution GI's take when smoking pot and the reluctance of their superior officers to report them when they are caught. Unless he's a rabidly gung-ho type, the commanding officer thinks twice before sending up a man with whom he shares the kinship forged by the rigors of combat.

Military officials estimate that one out of every two hundred GI's in Vietnam has smoked pot at least once. GI opinion puts this figure much higher. Of ninety-five inmates questioned in the Long Binh stockade in 1967, seventy-nine admitted having smoked pot. Ten percent indicated they had their first smoke in the military; forty-five percent had smoked before heeding Uncle Sam's call to duty; and the remaining forty-five percent began the practice in Vietnam. With the pot habit spreading throughout the United States, these figures are not surprising.

The CID agents and MP's alike have responded to this challenge by intensifying their preparedness to detect pot in military quarters. Before being sent to Vietnam, the agents now take a refresher course in drugs sponsored by the Federal Bureau of Narcotics at the Berkeley campus of UCLA. Most MP's are taught to smell and otherwise establish the presence of marijuana. But since many of them turn on themselves, they tend to be casual about finding pot smokers except in cases where the violation is glaringly obvious.

Attempts to strangle the supply at the source—that of the Vietnamese pushers—is hamstrung by the fact that this is the province of the Vietnamese police. By the time a raid has been planned and coordinated between the two authorities, the Vietnamese suspect, more often than not, has flown the coop. It's no wonder that the American law enforcers have long been suspicious of the link between the Vietnamese police and the pushers.

Servicemen are quick to point out that it is relatively easy to obtain "speed," i.e. amphetamines (which are potentially more harmful to the body than smoking pot) from the medic's supply room, if the soldier says that he needs to stay awake or requires extra energy for a tough mission. They say that since the military authorities do not care what happens to the GI's body as long as it functions in the line of duty, marijuana should be scrapped from the list of offenses.

Rarely does an offense result in a general court-martial, the outcome of which is certain to be five years at hard labor and a dishonorable discharge. The offender in Vietnam is usually tried by a special court that will most likely sentence him to six months in the stockade and forfeiture of pay.

Such lenience is, perhaps, partly to be explained by the military's unstated awareness that smoking marijuana does, in some cases, give a lift to lonely, frightened, or disheartened soldiers who are fighting an unpopular war thousands of miles from home.

One twenty-one-year old Pfc., who is never to be found without a pack of joints, claims that "You just couldn't fight if you didn't have any pot. You wouldn't be of any use because you'd be too scared. The NCO's and the officers know that and they don't hassle us about it."

Marijuana found on dead and wounded GI's supplies ample evidence that smoking takes place under combat conditions. Prosecution of a severely mangled serviceman would no doubt be looked upon as carrying the enforcement of discipline to absurd lengths.

The American authorities are, however, very serious about pot sent through the mail from Vietnam. Some GI's stationed in rear-line posts such as Saigon have made this practically a full-time occupation, salting away a sizeable nest egg by the time their tour of duty is up. Marijuana from Vietnam finds it way across the Pacific stuffed in souvenirs, baggage, and footlockers. It's impossible for the Army Post Office inspectors to check even a fraction of the tons of mail being sent home by half-a-million men. One sergeant, a habitual smoker, admitted to having stocked up on enough pot back home to last him several years. A number of arrests have been made, however.

Changes come slowly in the military establishment, but the generations now fighting the war in Vietnam may well be influential. It will take many years before their impact will be felt. No doubt, young soldiers, having smoked pot and liked it, are thinking of ways to combat the old bugaboos.

SECTION TWO:

LSD

CHAPTER ELEVEN

THE FIRST TRIP: BLAZING THE PSYCHEDELIC TRAIL

A Bicycle Ride, Waltzing Mice, and Schizophrenia

Thirty years have passed since a gangling Swiss chemist first synthesized the drug that is hailed from hippie crash pads as man's savior, hedged by psychiatrists as a possible therapeutic aid—and denounced by the nation's keepers as a mind-warping compound that threatens to turn America into a country of starry-eyed zombies.

No outcry signaled the unassuming beginnings of lysergic acid dyethylamide in the spring of 1938. In a cloistered laboratory of the Sandoz Chemical Works, just outside Basel, Switzerland, Dr. Albert Hoffman, a chemist and deputy director of the company, and his assistant, Dr. Arthur Stoll, were experimenting with synthesizations of a number of ergot-related compounds. At the time, the firm was already marketing several such derivatives as inducements to uterine contractions after childbirth.

Even before it became in 1935 the base of a number of drugs used mainly in after-birth care and migraine treatment, ergot had a remarkable history in the archives of European medicine. A parasitic fungus that once flourished in rye fields became the scourge of European peasants. They knew it as a substance that caused a gangrenous numbness and blackening of extremities and convulsions—a disease they called St. Anthony's fire. Before the intervention of a slow and painful death, the victim's toes and fingers would turn so brittle that they dropped from the body like leaves from a tree. Prayers to St. Anthony for deliverance from this "holy fire" were in vain.

There was, however, another face to *Claviceps purpurea,* as the diseased kernels of rye are medically known. Locked inside the husks was a veritable chemical factory with a number of beneficial properties. European midwives had long depended on these qualities to assist in childbirth and even in the performance of abortions, which the constrictive qualities of ergot aided by limiting excessive bleeding.

Another side effect, which was to prove important in Dr. Hoffman's experiments centuries later, were the visual and mental aberrations following the ingestion of the spoiled rye flour. It is now known that lysergic acid is one of the related parts or constituents characteristic of the ergot alkaloids.

Dr. Hoffman and his assistant were innocently searching for a useful combination of chemical tourniquet and analeptic. He called the resulting compound LSD-25 because it was discovered during the twenty-fifth experiment in a series of ergot tests.

The next five years of the newly synthesized drug were uneventful. The most powerful mind-expanding compound in nature's storeroom sat on the shelf of the Sandoz Chemical Works until April 16, 1943.

On the balmy spring afternoon of that day the war convulsing Europe seemed remote to the dark-haired chemist pedaling home on his bicycle along the road leading out of Basel. The road wound through picture-postcard scenery of towering mountains bathed in sunlight. Waterfalls ran from snowcaps into the surging countryside that was alive with birdcalls and the echôes of bells tinkling from the necks of grazing cows. But that day his ride was marred by increasingly pronounced feelings of discomfort and dizziness. Unknown to himself at the time, he was on his first "acid trip." His laboratory report of the day included the following account.

> Last Friday on the 16th of April I had to leave my work in the laboratory and go home because I felt strangely restless and dizzy. I got home, lay down and sank into a not unpleasant delirium which was characterized by an extreme degree of fantasy (a kind of trance). I kept my eyes closed because I found the daylight very unpleasant. Fantastic visions of extraordinary vividness accompanied by a kaleidoscopic-like play of intense colora-

tion continuously swirled around my head. The condition lasted for about two hours.*

Unable to explain the symptoms, Hoffman decided to experiment upon himself. He proceeded cautiously, swallowing 250 micrograms, a very small dose by any other standards, but at least two-and-a-half times the amount now considered proper, and ten times the dosage needed to produce hallucinations.

The minute particle—one-millionth of an ounce—took effect half an hour later. Nervousness and sensations of dizziness alternated with sudden spells of laughter. He felt unable to concentrate on his work. In recording the effects, he got as far as noting the fact that his vision was distorted. At that point he succumbed completely to the impact of the first dose of LSD consciously administered to the human body. He wrote later:

> The last words were written only with great difficulty. I had asked my laboratory assistant to accompany me home since I assumed the situation would progress in a manner similar to last Friday. But on the way home (on a bicycle since no other vehicle was available because of the war) the symptoms developed into a much greater intensity than the first time. I had the greatest difficulty in speaking coherently and my field of vision fluctuated and was distorted like the reflections in an amusement park mirror. I also had the impression that I was hardly moving. Later my assistant told me that I was pedalling at a good speed.

This description is the first and only account by a trained observer in which the subject had no preconception of what could be expected to happen. The setting, as Dr. Leary would term it later, was as close to zero as it is ever likely to be. Hoffman's condition intensified until he could barely communicate. He continues in his notebook:

> So far as I can remember the high point of the crisis had passed by the time the doctor arrived. It was characterized by the symptoms of dizziness, visual distortion, the faces of those present appeared like grotesque colored masks, strong agitation alternating with paresis, the head, body and extremities sometimes cold and numb; a metallic taste on the tongue; throat dry and shrivelled; feeling of suffocation; confusion alternating with a clear appreciation of the situation; at times standing outside myself as

*From The Swiss Archives of Neurology, Vol. 60, p. 279.

a neutral observer and hearing myself muttering jargon and screaming half-madly.

The doctor found a somewhat weak pulse but in general a normal circulation. Six hours after taking the drug my situation had improved definitely. The perceptual distortions were still present—everything seemed to undulate and their proportions were distorted like the reflections on a choppy water surface. Everything was changing with unpleasant, predominantly poisonous green and blue color tones. With closed eyes multi-hued metamorphosizing fantastic images overwhelmed me, especially noteworthy was the fact that sounds were transposed into visual sensations so that from each tone or noise a horrible color picture was evoked changing in form and color kaleidoscopically.

Dr. Hoffman's slender account was the first of more than four thousand articles that have since covered every aspect of the LSD experience. More information, however, about this new compound that seemingly influenced the brain metabolism of man was slow in coming, for Dr. Hoffman's discovery had fired the imagination of but a handful of scientists. Then, in 1947, five years later, the real breakthrough came. The doctor, who had been working with volunteers from other Sandoz laboratories, passed some LSD-25 on to a medical doctor and psychiatrist in Zurich—Dr. W. A. Stoll, the son of the chemist who had originally helped him prepare the first known batch of LSD in 1938.

At that time Dr. Stoll operated a psychiatric clinic at Zurich University, where he administered the LSD to both normal volunteers and some mental patients. Giving modest doses of the drug to fifteen normal volunteers, he confirmed in detail the reactions Hoffman had already reported. He also verified that hallucinatory reactions followed the administering of as little as thirty micrograms of LSD. Stoll's evidence and reports subsequently opened the doors to further LSD tests in Germany, Scandinavia, and other European laboratories—all separate efforts that added to the growing lore of the drug.

The first LSD was shipped to the United States in 1949. It was sent to the late psychiatrist, Dr. Max Rinkel of the Massachusetts Mental Health Center, who administered it to over one hundred volunteers and confirmed the results of the European researchers. To a man, the psychiatrists were struck by the parallel between LSD-influenced subjects and the delusions of schizophrenics. Dr. Rinkel's similar findings set the medical world astir. Could it be that nature's pharmacopoeia had finally yielded a catalyst for imitation psychoses that would be helpful in understanding the mechanism of the disorder? This was one of the first questions thrown into the ring of medical research.

Experiments on animals yielded further insights into this dramatic discovery, though too many unknowns still remained. What happened to the drug in the body? How much of the drug would kill? What were its cumulative effects? Even today LSD's role in mental therapy is still largely uncharted.

At the beginning of the fifties, pharmacologists were giving the drug to every type of laboratory animal. They even fed it to some animals not ordinarily used for research purposes in order to substantiate their findings with the most unequivocal evidence. The same physiological effects—dilation of the pupil, pilo-erection (the furred equivalent of goose bumps on humans), increased body temperature, and a rise in blood sugar—that had been observed in human volunteers were also clearly displayed by the animals dosed with the drug.

Aside from the body changes, however, there were a number of other unaccountable reactions. Under the influence of LSD, spiders built more perfect and elaborate webs. Some animals became more passive. Rats placed on a level surface acted as if they were scaling an incline. They became extremely agitated and hugged the level surface as if they were about to fall off. LSD given to waltzing mice agitated the rodents so much that they stopped dancing. Goats used in the experiments walked about in compulsive patterns, such as squares, figure eights, ovals, circles, retracing their steps over and over like nervous expectant fathers.

One of the most spectacular tests was run by Dr. Louis West, a psychiatrist at the University of Oklahoma. In an attempt to duplicate recurring musth—a periodic madness suffered by elephants—he used an air pistol to shoot an elephant in the Oklahoma City Zoo from a range of twenty-five feet with about three hundred thousand micrograms of LSD (one thousand times the average human dose). The seven-thousand-pound animal failed to go into the furies expected. Instead it collapsed in the throes of spasmodic seizures and died. It might have succumbed to suffocation caused by spasms closing the throat, or it is possible that the syringe had penetrated a vein, thus speeding up the unexpected effects and causing the elephant to lapse into its seizure. Similar experiments carried out on cats, employing twice the normal amount of LSD and sometimes injected directly into the veins, did not yield lethal results. What, then, is the lethal dose?

Researchers have discovered they need an extremely large amount of LSD to cause death to an animal. The chief of pharmacology at Sandoz' laboratory, Dr. Ernst Rothlin, found that on a weight-to-weight basis with humans he had to inject twenty thousand times the normal dose into the veins of mice to kill them; five thousand times the normal dose, to kill rats; and one hundred times the normal dose, to kill rabbits. Dr. Rothlin thinks the oversized doses of LSD kill the animals by depressing their brain's breathing center, which simply stops functioning. Currently, the dose lethal to humans is not known.

There were some other interesting behavioral effects in the animal experiments. Carp, a species of fish notably resistant to most other drugs, dramatically changed their way of living. Dr. Howard A. Loeb, a biologist at the New York State Conservation Department, experimented on fifteen two-pound carp by dosing their water with one part LSD to one-millionth part water. Carp are bottom fish and seldom swim to the water's surface. Under the influence of LSD, however, they immediately broke the water line with their noses pointed skyward, hovering at the top of the tank and clustering together. They also showed a slight discoloration.

Do animals undergo hallucinations? Just as it would be virtually impossible to obtain the subjective reactions of the drug on a human unable to speak or communicate, it would be very difficult to determine the psychological changes in animals. As noted previously, animals do undergo the same dilation of pupils and rise in temperature that humans experience. A series of experiments has demonstrated that an animal under LSD will respond more rapidly to a weaker stimulus (noise or light) than will an untreated animal. This phenomenon indicates a lowering of the sensation threshold, comparable to the enhanced sensory perception in humans.

Further comparisons between the psychic effects in animals and humans cannot be made. The researchers had to experiment on man himself.

CHAPTER TWELVE

LSD FOR EVERYONE: THE LEARY-ALPERT COMPLEX

Dropouts Turn America On

No one person has done more to popularize the cult of LSD and its use around the world than handsome, blue-eyed, fiftyish former Harvard professor, Dr. Timothy Leary. The public has come to identify him almost exclusively with LSD. He has admitted to having taken more than five hundred "trips," a number that qualifies him as the drug's foremost theoretical expert, spokesman, and philosopher.

Whether he is a corrupter of youth or a saint—as opinion has either castigated or praised him—there is no denying that he has boldly preached the life-affirming qualities of LSD as opposed to what he considers man's drab, unenlightened condition in the drugless state. Almost single-handedly Leary has transformed LSD from a medical curiosity into one of the most controversial drugs since opium.

Leary's dedication has cost him dearly. Although his first two years at Harvard were relatively free of trouble, he has since trod a tortuous road. Dismissed from Harvard, arrested and charged twice with the possession of hallucinogens, run out of Boston and Mexico, scored by the medical profession and vilified in the public press, his only comfort has been a growing community of like-minded cultists and the knowledge that his crusade has made LSD a household word around the nation. His message has also caused nervous politicians to rush through legislation as a deterrent against the use of the drug. But, as today's evidence shows, it is a taboo more honored in the breach than in the observance.

Leary's early experiment with hallucinogens in Cuernavaca, Mexico, came at a time when the "kick" of marijuana was beginning to fade on college campuses. The LSD cult has grown steadily in universities over the years, promising its users "trips" to places no marijuana smoker had ever visited. Occasionally a student would "freak out" (have a bad experience with the drug), an incident that would immediately flare into headlines. The increasing concern over the drug by the media, clergy, and government authorities left no doubt: The LSD generation had come into existence.

The progenitor of this new breed of youth was born in 1920 in Springfield, Massachusetts, the only son of Irish Catholic parents. His father was a dentist and his youth was typical of an upper middle-class boy, although Leary now claims he was first turned on at the age of six with nitrous oxide (laughing gas) in his father's office.

He earned a degree in psychology at the University of Alabama followed by a Master's degree from Washington State University. He eventually took his Ph.D. in clinical psychology at the University of California in 1950. Afterward, he lectured at the Kaiser Foundation Hospital in Oakland, California, where he became Director of Psychological Research in 1953. It was here that he wrote a paper on personality diagnosis that later led to a post on the Harvard faculty.

Suddenly widowed and accompanied by his two children, he left his job and the United States and spent a few years wandering around the world and lecturing in Mexico, Spain, Italy, and Denmark. He was to settle down again in 1959 when, upon the urging of Dr. David McClelland, Director of Harvard's Center for Research in Personality, he accepted a post on his staff. During the first years at Harvard, he gave little evidence of the controversial nature he was to exhibit in future years. He went quietly about his work, collaborating on two textbooks on clinical psychology.

It was the summer of 1960, following his appointment at Harvard, that was to be the turning point in his life. Leary was on vacation in Mexico, lounging beside a pool at a friend's villa in Cuernavaca, when he heard about a certain species of mushroom that was rumored to cause far-reaching mental aberrations. Possessing the psychologist's interest in anything holding the power to affect the mind, Leary obtained some of these mushrooms (which contained psilocybin) from an old woman known as "Crazy Jane," who lived up in the mountains some miles from town. Back at the villa, he nibbled them by the edge of the swimming pool. Some years later he said of this first experience that he realized immediately that the old Timothy Leary was dead and "the Timothy Leary game" was over.

Returning to Harvard in the fall of 1960, he made his first convert to the hallucinogenic experience—a twenty-nine-year-old fellow faculty member, Dr. Richard Alpert, also on the staff of the Research Center. Together, they experimented further with hallucinogens, using first psilocybin, which had been synthesized from the magic mushrooms the year before. They also conferred with the late Aldous Huxley, then in residence at M.I.T.

Huxley, an early experimenter with hallucinogenic drugs, had written a book, *Doors of Perception,* published by Harper and Row in 1954, about the subject based on his experiences with mescaline. In an article written in 1958 for the *Saturday Evening Post,* Huxley spoke about "a chemical evangelism that would make it possible for large numbers of men and women to achieve a radical self-transcendence, and a deeper understanding of the nature of things. And this revival of religion will be at the same time a revolution." The scholarly Englishman shared the enthusiasm of the two teachers, and Leary and Alpert left with a new dedication to continue the experiments which, until that time, they had limited to themselves.

Later that fall, using psilocybin secured from the Sandoz Pharmaceuticals Company at Hanover, New Jersey—the American subsidiary of the Swiss chemical company that held patents on both psilocybin and LSD—Leary and Alpert began experiments on psychology students.

These first tentative probes were carried out with the approval of the Research Center. But trouble soon developed in January, 1959, when they began their first large-scale investigation of the effects of hallucinogens—a two-year pilot program involving thirty-five prisoners at the Massachusetts Correction Institution at Concord.

Their studies sought to determine if the mind-expanding properties of psychedelic drugs could provide the subjects with insights that would conclusively alter their criminal life. In carrying out their research, however, they challenged a primary principle of scientific research—that the researcher should at all costs avoid participating in the experiment and maintain an objective attitude throughout. Interaction between the subject and researcher, however, was one of Huxley's cardinal rules. He believed that, in the impersonal setting of the clinic, the psychedelic experience could do more harm than good. Leary and Alpert, therefore, avoided approaching their convict patients at Concord prison as human guinea pigs and, instead, chose to set up a friendly relationship of mutual respect.

Out of these experiments came a report comparing the history of treated prisoners after release with the records of those who had not been given the Harvard cure. Although it showed that a higher percentage of the treated convicts managed to stay out of the courts and prisons of Massachusetts, their conclusions were not greeted with hosannas of praise in medical circles.

The conflict between the medical and personal use of hallucinogens was to become exacerbated in the years to follow. Although at first a medical doctor had been on hand for the prison experiments, subsequent work by the two psychologists did sometimes neglect such supervision.

Believing that the clinical surroundings somehow spoiled the true value of the drug experience, Leary began to hold sessions at home by candlelight and with the appropriate music. Gradually word spread around the Harvard campus that the two professors were in favor of the free use of hallucinogens, and by spring of 1961 certain Harvard officials showed their annoyance. It grew when a freshman, gathering information for a term paper, reported Leary as saying, "These things are great—just great," a comment that increased the misgivings of the officials about the spirit in which the experiments were carried out.

Reports of students securing LSD and other hallucinogens with the backing of Leary and Alpert appeared in the *Harvard Crimson,* the campus newspaper. In one of their psychology courses a number of students had asked for and received psilocybin for use in an experiment.

"We began to run more and more sessions with the drug, and students were involved," Alpert told an interviewer a few years later.

In spite of a promise secured by officials of the University Health Service in October, 1961, that the two professors would not use the drugs in experiments with undergraduates, hallucinogens were becoming increasingly popular at Harvard. Leary himself admitted that he continued to administer psilocybin to some four hundred volunteers between 1961 and 1963.

On March 14, 1962, an open attack came from the Center for Research in Personality. Dr. Herbert Kelman, a lecturer in social psychology in the department, challenged the Leary-Alpert method and concept of experimentation, branding it as being contrary to the whole tradition of psychological research.

"I question whether this project is carried out primarily as an intellectual endeavor, or whether it is being pursued as a new kind of experience to offer an answer to man's ills," he said.

The *Boston Herald* and media around the country spread word of this confrontation across the nation, prompting a joint investigation by the state and the Food and Drug Administration, which had jurisdiction over hallucinogenic drugs. Leary and Alpert were warned that under Massachusetts law they could not administer potentially harmful drugs unless a licensed medical doctor was present; students were again warned not to become involved in the experimentation and use of psychedelics. University officials also attempted to take the drugs out of the hands of the two professors.

Because of this harassment, they moved their drug operations completely off campus, setting up two groups outside of Boston for further studies of mind expansion. Alpert said, "Tim and I got depressed. This was the hottest thing that we ever were involved in and these people kept putting obstacles in our path."

The hostile Boston setting that summer forced Leary to return to Mexico, where he made tentative arrangements to rent an empty resort hotel in the town of Zihuatenejo on the Pacific Coast, about two hundred miles north of Acapulco.

When Leary and Alpert returned to Harvard in September of 1962, they announced the formation of their International Foundation for Internal Freedom (IFIF). Public reports at the time described Leary as a "madman" and an "addict" who was "trying to drive all those around him mad." All the publicity showered on LSD succeeded only in creating a growing underground movement that included intellectuals, students, and hippie groups across the nation. The *Harvard Crimson* reported psilocybin parties on campus, and LSD sugar cubes were going for as little as one dollar each.

In May of 1963 the Harvard establishment dropped its academic ax. Leary and Alpert were fired from their posts after an undergraduate had admitted to the dean that he had taken one of the drugs under the auspices of Dr. Alpert. Leary was fired shortly afterward on the technicality that he did not appear as scheduled for classes.

"It tears my heart to see what's happened to them," said McClelland, their mentor at Harvard. "They started out as good, sound scientists and now they've become cultists."

"These drugs apparently cause panic and temporary insanity in many officials who have not taken them," said Leary as he and Alpert fired off a joint declaration to the *Harvard Review*:

> Must we continue to jail, execute, exile our ecstatic visionaries, and then enshrine them as tomorrow's heroes? . . . Society needs educated priest-scholars to provide structure—the intellectual muscle, bone and skin to keep things together . . . The nervous system can be changed, integrated, recircuited, expanded in its function. These possibilities naturally threaten every branch of the Establishment . . . Our favorite concepts are standing in the way of a floodtide, two billion years building up. The verbal dam is collapsing. Head for the hills, or prepare your intellectual craft to flow with the current.

After Leary's dismissal from Harvard, the International Foundation for Internal Freedom found new headquarters in the hotel he had rented the previous summer. His Mexican experiments had a short but spectacular career, enduring all of six weeks before he was expelled from the country. While it lasted, the experimental community was deluged with applicants, including psychologists, psychiatrists, stockbrokers, actors and actresses from Hollywood, writers, and a yogi. More than five thousand Americans applied for the two-week sessions at the rate of one hundred dollars per week for bed and board and six dollars per dose of LSD—more applicants than it could handle. The project also attracted some hippie types who, after being refused admittance, set up lean-tos and tents near the hotel where they lounged around smoking marijuana.

All of these activities did not help the organization's reputation with the local authorities who had been further aroused by some other unfortunate events. One of Leary's guests had freaked out after having experienced his first dose of LSD and eventually ended up spending four days in a hospital in Mexico City. Another guest reportedly fell down a flight of stairs, injuring an eye and his head, and was forced to return to California, where he spent several months under psychiatric care. These incidents, fanned by rumors of the hotel's strange guests who were said to engage in all-night orgies and other debauches were breathlessly reported by the Mexican and American press.

Despite the furor, no strong impetus for deportation developed until Leary himself set into motion the apparatus that was to propel him out of Mexico. Again it was the result of the ever-widening split between Leary's views about the uses of LSD and those held by the medical profession. Accepting an invitation to read a paper on LSD before a group of doctors at the University of Mexico's Medical-Biological Institute, Leary outraged the director who found his message "very confused and valueless." At his behest the Mexican authorities investigated the Hotel Catalina retreat.

Leary and his followers were subsequently asked to leave the country within five days on the charge that they "had entered the country as tourists and were now engaged in unauthorized activities." Leary's defense of his center as a haven for "philosophers, educators, teachers, and intellectuals devoted to a new movement of internal liberation" failed to convince the Mexican authorities.

The Mexican fiasco and the national publicity that grew out of it actually aided the growth of the LSD cult. By the fall of 1963 most of the major national magazines had done feature stories on Leary and/or LSD. Use of LSD, previously limited to small groups of intellectuals and college students, was now becoming a mass movement as Leary continued his crusade from a new locale—the Millbrook estate in upstate New York. Here he created a new organization called the Castalia Foundation to replace the now-dead IFIF.

The Castalia Foundation's home was a rented four-thousand-acre estate in Duchess County, New York, which included a rambling baroque sixty-four-room mansion. From these headquarters Leary threw himself full time into the promotion of LSD as the universal experience. Since use of the drug in the United States was not permitted, Leary announced that ego transcendence could be accomplished without the use of artificial compounds. His group at Millbrook, he claimed, was achieving this state through the use of meditation, setting, and other nondrug devices.

The methods used at Millbrook, he said, "involved yoga-like breathing exercises, stroboscopic light projections on the ceiling, and the use of psychedelic music." He did not, however, categorically deny that LSD was never being used.

Early in 1966 Leary sprang into the nation's headlines again when he was arrested for transporting marijuana into this country from Mexico. The glare of publicity was once more cast upon him. After he admitted, during his trial, to occasionally smoking marijuana, United States District Judge Ben Connally in March of 1966 imposed the stiffest penalty the law allowed—a forty-thousand-dollar fine and five-to-thirty years in the penitentiary (a conviction that has since been overturned by the Supreme Court, as previously noted).

More trouble followed. About a month later, on April 17, 1966, a raiding party of thirty men led by Duchess County District Attorney John Heilman, and Sheriff Lawrence Quinlan, burst into Millbrook's Castalia Foundation. Before dragging Leary off to jail for the second time in a little more than a month, the police spent five hours searching the establishment while the former Harvard professor, wearing only his pajama tops, and about twenty other members of his party were required to stand by and watch. Also present that night were Leary's sixteen-year-old son, three other teen-agers, and five young children.

The search party reported it had found a bag of marijuana on the premises. Leary, however, denied knowledge of any illegal drugs in the mansion.

Explaining the events to a young woman reporter some time after the incident, he asked her, "My dear, you don't expect that thirty policemen could search this house for five hours *without* finding marijuana, do you?"

The county officials stated that they had been watching the house for weeks. Sheriff Quinlan said the raid was ordered only after his men "had observed people acting differently." He claimed they had seen "a great many people dancing wildly around a bonfire, and that's not normal."

The police were also shocked at finding "men and women sleeping together in several rooms on mattresses out on the floor itself."

The Castalia Foundation director explained the lack of furniture as being "more natural" than a house cluttered with unnecessary accouterments. He was also outraged by the police asking the guests such questions as whether they had engaged in sexual intercourse while staying at the house.

Leary believes he is being harassed by the law enforcement agencies and that his civil rights are being stepped on with impunity and on the vaguest of charges.

"They are trampling on my civil liberties," he declared on the occasion of the arrest, denying any orgiastic occurrences at Millbrook that weekend. He explained that all of the action on the estate had been confined to "some tree chopping, some singing around a campfire and listening to recordings."

Leary's next move took his disciples by surprise. Shortly after his second arrest he appeared at New York City's Town Hall and delivered a two-hour lecture to an audience of eight hundred of his followers in which he called for a one-year moratorium on the use of hallucinogens. He spoke about the five ascending levels of consciousness that had led him to a point where he claimed to be able to see not only his own conception nine months before he was born, but even farther back to the chain of DNA molecules that holds all the hereditary properties passed down through the ages of man and animals preceding him.

The five levels, according to Leary, are: (1) that of alcohol and narcotics, an inhibiting and limiting level of consciousness; (2) that of the normal everyday vision of the external world, a surface level of consciousness; (3) the level of marijuana, which is a mild hallucinogen pertaining to the level of sensory-consciousness; (4) the level of the LSD-induced states; (5) and, finally, "that peculiar flash for which we have no word but which I'll call 'soul.' "

During 1966 he appeared before three different Congressional committees investigating the use of LSD and other related drugs. The testimony he gave before each of these committees was substantially the same. He said that LSD had been misunderstood and that his statements about the drug were misunderstood; and that even if legislation banned the drug, it would be flouted by the new generation, which was unanimously in favor of its use.

Citing the need for greater understanding of the effects of LSD as opposed to laws prohibiting its use, he revealed having taken LSD himself more than five hundred times and having given it to others who wanted it. He drew a parallel to the Volstead Act of the twenties, which, besides failing to eliminate the consumption of alcohol, had actually brought about a lowering of the standards of the quality of the product and gangster control of its manufacture. A ban on LSD, he predicted, would produce similar results.

He suggested that colleges be authorized to conduct laboratory courses in LSD. At the same time, he agreed that legislators might institute a general ban on LSD except in legalized psychedelic centers to be operated under government license.

Soon after, a vocal minority of youngsters expressed their disappointment in what they considered to be an about-face in Leary's former intransigent position. It was probably this consideration that impelled their leader to change his mind again, and once more advocate the unrestrained use of LSD.

The picture as it stands today is as fluid as it has been in the past. The battle of the LSD advocates and the legal artillery ranged against them continues to rage mainly because of the confusion in both camps. Its decisive outcome will depend to a great extent on the public.

CHAPTER THIRTEEN

THE NEW PROHIBITION: ANTI-LSD LEGISLATION

The Establishment Versus Flower Power

Pressure for restrictive legislation has slowly been building up. A good many scientists look askance at this development. They argue that, while hippies and college students can easily obtain LSD on the black market, they are limited to legitimate sources. Restrictive legislation would, in the scientific view, seriously hamper further constructive research on the application of LSD to specific medical problems. Testifying before Senate investigating committees, they urged the lawmakers to be moderate.

"It has not been proven that LSD is actually helpful in treating mental disorders, but it is known that it can be harmful to humans," said Dr. Gerald Klee, an authority on drugs, adding, "It does not follow, however, that we should abandon all clinical investigations with this drug. It is necessary to experiment with new types of treatment even if it involves taking calculated risks if we are ever to achieve greater success in treating patients."

The slow and painstaking efforts made by clinical researchers, however, were overshadowed by the pop cult established by Leary. Reports of hallucinatory visions, trips within the mind, debauchery, and mental breakdown quashed the doctors' quiet rational arguments for continued freedom in the use of LSD for research. Leary, of course, was also against restrictive legislation, but he advocated complete freedom of use.

The argument against the drug, as one psychologist pointed out, was not so much its possible danger (there had been no incident of harm to a user of LSD at the time), but that it went against an ingrained puritanical ethic. Most of the supporters of LSD described it as nonaddictive and unlikely to cause harmful side effects in most subjects. The idea of gaining pleasure from a drug without compensatory harm frightens the authorities because it is not consistent with our puritanical ethics, they claimed.

As Leary himself pointed out, "Americans drink more alcohol and swallow more pep and sleeping pills per capita than any other people in the world. However, the psychology that follows these drugs is not that they give pleasure, but that they are practical tools for regulating the body."

The investigations into LSD picked up steam with the case of a medical school dropout who had allegedly stabbed to death his mother-in-law in her Brooklyn apartment.

Harvard-graduate Steven Kessler had carried out experiments with psychedelic drugs before quitting his medical studies at the University of the State of New York. On one occasion, he had been admitted to Bellevue Hospital with a panic reaction to a dose of hallucinogens. Separated from his wife at the time of the murder, Kessler had no job and was not attending any school.

The exact facts about the case are not clear. One Monday, he went in search of his wife at the home of his mother-in-law, Florence Cooper, who told him that she was not there. He got into some sort of argument and she telephoned her husband. When her husband arrived home later that day, he found his wife dead, her throat slit and a dozen stab wounds in her chest. The police found Kessler at home two hours later, taking a shower.

They quoted the suspect as saying, "Did I kill my wife? Did I rape anybody? What have I done? Man, I've been flying for three days on LSD."

Three days later when Kessler was arraigned in Brooklyn Court, he wept and pleaded to the judge, "Will you please put me back in Bellevue? Please. I don't know what happened. If I did, I would be much happier."

When the case was brought to court, the New York press tagged the proceedings the "LSD Murder Trial." Kessler's lawyer maintained that his client, an admitted LSD user, had been in a state of "amnesia" at the time, and that he was not responsible for his actions.

Kessler, testifying on his own behalf, admitted taking LSD five times but said the last time had been in 1966, one month before Mrs. Cooper's death. Other witnesses, however, testified that Kessler had admitted to them that he took LSD three times on the weekend of the murder—Friday, Sunday, and Monday, only hours before Mrs. Cooper was killed on April 11. Also brought into evidence was Kessler's statement to arresting officers that he had been "flying on LSD" for three days.

The defense, however, continued to stick to its contention that Kessler had been "in a state of complete amnesia" at the time of the murder and could not be held accountable for the charge against him. It did not try to prove that this was due to LSD.

The prosecution, based on the testimony of various doctors, including Dr. Walter Bromberg, Head of Criminal Psychiatry at King's County Hospital in Brooklyn where Kessler was committed after his arrest, maintained that the accused was in control of his faculties when he committed the murder and was aware of the consequences. Dr. Bromberg testified that he had treated fifteen patients with LSD and all had been aware of their surroundings and of the drug's influence.

He went on to state that, "Three days is a long time to be high on LSD—not that it can't be done—but he would have to take some massive doses on the second and third days. I would say it is doubtful that the murder can be attributed to LSD. With the man's mental background and the massive dose on the third day, I suppose it is remotely possible. My only further comment would be that it would seem fair to investigate the possibility and the man's story before terming it an LSD murder—which I saw in some of the papers."

Whether it was an LSD murder or not, it did prompt the New York State Legislature to consider two bills calling for prison sentences of up to twenty years for those convicted of selling or giving away LSD. The federal and state governments, as well as law-enforcement agencies around the country, thereafter came under increasing pressure to pass extremely punitive legislation.

Another case in New York City involved a child who "went mad" after accidentally swallowing a dose of LSD that her eighteen-year-old uncle had purchased in Greenwich Village and had left in the refrigerator.

Donna Wingemothe, a five-year-old Brooklyn girl, alternately laughing and screaming hysterically, was taken to a hospital where her stomach was pumped. She was released three days later, without any apparent aftereffects. Several doctors stated, however, that pumping the child's stomach was a waste of time since LSD disappears into the blood almost immediately.

There were many other such reports. One involved two children in Chicago who accidentally swallowed LSD and were rushed to a hospital in what was called a "critical" condition. Both recovered quickly. A young high school coed in Sherman Oaks, California, was found unconscious on a street corner. Police attributed her state to LSD. Another case involved a Harvard student left helpless for four days during which time he became convinced that he was only six inches tall. There was the Long Island couple hospitalized for psychiatric treatment because the husband thought he was Christ and the wife believed him. A woman in Los Angeles ripped off her clothes and ran naked through the streets looking for absolution for imagined sins. Dozens of other reports can be added to these cases.

Against this background no less than three United States Senate subcommittees were busy investigating LSD. They heard testimony from authorities stating that LSD had precipitated a crisis. They heard some experts say that LSD is bad while other experts declared that LSD is beneficial. At the same time, they continued to pass more restrictive legislation, the most important of which was the Drug Abuse Control Amendment Act to change the basic Federal Food, Drug and Cosmetics Act (Bill No. 89-74).

This spate of legislative activity constituted the initial federal controls of black-market LSD. They were signed into law by President Johnson on July 15, 1965, although they did not become effective for seven months—until February 1, 1966. The Drug Abuse Control Amendment Act of 1965 grouped depressants, stimulants, and hallucinogenic drugs under one heading, and made manufacture, processing, distribution, or sale of such items a federal offense punishable by up to one year in jail and a thousand-dollar fine.

The penalty is stricter in cases where the drug is sold to persons under twenty-one years of age. In these instances, the penalty of conviction is up to two years in jail and a five-thousand-dollar fine for the first offense, and up to six years in jail and a fifteen-thousand-dollar fine for subsequent convictions. Other hallucinogens besides LSD included in this law were dimethyltryptamine (DMT), mescaline, peyote, psilocybin, and psilocin.

The law, however, exempted peyote as used in the official ceremonies of the Native American Church, although it stipulated that the congregationalists in this Indian religious organization must register with the government and keep accurate records. By giving legal sanction to the drug used by this group (incorporated sixty years ago as a Christian church) as a sacrament in its rituals, the government opened a loophole for less venerable religious establishments, such as Timothy Leary's League for Spiritual Discovery which has as its avowed basic and only tenet the ritualistic use of psychochemicals.

Although the law did not make possession of LSD itself illegal, some state legislatures began taking action in this direction. In New York, public-health laws were instituted to make possession of LSD a misdemeanor for the first offender; sale of the drug was judged a felony with a maximum of a two-year jail sentence.

The law states: "The possession, sale, exchange, or giving away of hallucinogenic drugs or preparations by other than registered manufacturers or licensed physicians who hold a license issued by the Commission of Mental Hygiene to receive such drugs shall constitute a violation."

Convictions carry penalties of up to one year in jail and a five-hundred-dollar fine for a first offense, and two years in jail and a thousand-dollar fine for subsequent convictions.

In California, a law was passed in May, 1966, that made unauthorized possession of LSD a misdemeanor punishable by a maximum fine of a thousand dollars or a year in jail; unauthorized manufacture or possession for the purpose of sale of the drug constitute a felony punishable by one to five years in jail for the first offense, and two to ten years for the second offense.

This legislation was opposed by clergy, educators, and hippies, all of whom disliked to see the LSD user branded as a criminal. But a massive campaign by the state attorney general, the governor, and a group of determined legislators managed to carry the bill through.

Meanwhile, the Federal Food and Drug Administration had sent out warnings of the LSD menace to all drug manufacturers with the result that the only legal manufacturer of the compound pulled the drug off the experimental market.

Legislation, however, did produce a reaction from the researchers, who seemed to be the only people hurt by the massive crackdown. A number of their programs were stranded when the government ruling shut off the supply from the manufacturers. Said one serious medical investigator: "It seems as though medical scientists are the only ones who have any trouble getting LSD these days. Anybody else who wants it can obtain it from the black market."

Most doctors blame the mass media for distorting the nature of LSD, claiming that they only emphasized its dangers. None of the stories, they say, ever mentioned any of its more beneficial properties brought to light by medical research.

As the legal clamps were tightened, Leary and Alpert kept up their campaign against the restrictive laws with unabated intensity. Leary's followers, along with two other groups based in Florida and Arizona, felt that LSD should be legally sanctioned for use by organizations with mystical and religious intentions. Their demands asked for an exemptive status similar to that of the Native American Church, which, as noted earlier, was allowed by law to use peyote in its religious services.

"It is to be hoped," said Alpert, "that our vision and our commitments to growth of the individual and society will prevent us from legislating out of existence one of man's greatest chances to expand the boundaries of his mind, his individuality, and his culture."

Leary's impassioned testimony had little effect on one of the Senate subcommittees before which he was invited to state the LSD case. He argued that the prohibitive legislation would give rise to a black market whose lack of quality control would increase the danger of using the drug. The legislation itself, he implied, would not stop the so-called "LSD crisis," and he contended that "millions will be using LSD by 1970; more are turning on, every day." He proposed the establishment of a Commission of Psychochemical Education, which, in his words, would be a "blue-ribbon panel of neurologists, pharmacologists, psychologists, educators, and religious leaders who will survey the entire field of psychochemical research."

The reaction of "acidheads" to the initial LSD laws was unexpectedly mild, possibly because they had no trouble obtaining the drug in the underground market. Students could be seen wearing buttons reading, "Support your local travel agent," and "Fly now—Pay later."

The latest legislation against hallucinogens is likely to make use and sale of the drug more hazardous. Increasing the penalties imposed by the Drug Abuse Control Amendment Act of 1965, a new bill signed by President Johnson on October 25, 1968, raised manufacture, sale, and distribution of LSD and other hallucinogens from a misdemeanor to a felony punishable by five years imprisonment and a ten-thousand-dollar fine. Illegal possession of the drug was made a misdemeanor with a maximum penalty of one year and a thousand-dollar fine.

The acidheads stay cool. As one campus hippie said, "No matter what the Establishment does, we'll always be able to get acid. What can they do to stop us? It's easy to manufacture. The user never has any hang-ups about needing it and only if you're real dumb do you get busted. Besides, its illegality will only make it more exotic and sought after by those who have not tried it yet."

CHAPTER FOURTEEN

BLACK-MARKET ACID: THE THREAT OF THE MAFIA

Cornering the Underground Acid Market

The campus hippie was not alone in his challenge. A doctor testifying before one of the Senate investigating committees, stated that "LSD is apparently so easy to manufacture that it is hard to see how policing can handle the problem."

The drug isn't just easy to manufacture, but it is almost impossible to detect, quite easy to distribute, and used by a segment of society that the police cannot easily patrol.

First of all, LSD is colorless, odorless, and only one ounce is enough to "book" three hundred thousand trips. It has been distributed as virtually undetectable powder on facial tissue, on the back of postage stamps, in handkerchiefs, or on any article of clothing that will absorb the acid. Nobody uses sugar cubes any more except as decoys.

Students vacationing in Europe have brought thousands of acid trips back to the United States in packs of cigarettes, in the chambers of fountain pens, absorbed in the pages of a book, the shoelace of a sneaker, or in any other object usually worn or carried by the traveler.

When the East Coast Customs Office was questioned about acid smuggling from Europe, they claimed not to know of any such operation, which only indicated that it was hardly detectable. The Food and Drug Administration agents readily admitted that plenty of clandestine acid enters the United States, as the numerous raids of distributors in this country have shown.

The problem of enforcing the anti-LSD laws put on the books is therefore a difficult task. The federal undercover agent finds it difficult to determine just what it is he bought or confiscated. Acid in powder form appears white, and in solution is indistinguishable from water (except where an individual manufacturer tints his solution as a mark of quality or as a method to measure its varying strengths for dilution purposes).

Another problem that arose was the discovery and marketing of new hallucinogens, such as STP. Because of the time lag between its discovery and the propulsion required to set the legal mechanism in motion, it was possible for a time to sell STP with relative freedom and quite legally.

The task of enforcing the new anti-LSD laws at first went to agents of the Food and Drug Administration, a group of people who were completely unfamiliar with the properties and chemical characteristics of the psychedelics. The FDA men were more at home poking around in drug factories to check out illegalities in industrial practices. Although the investigators didn't even have a positive test for LSD prior to 1966, the drug-control amendments of 1965 were further altered a year later to give greater powers to the Food and Drug Administration. Under the Bureau of Drug Abuse Control—an enforcement agency for monitoring the laws of the FDA set up in 1966—they had jurisdiction not only over black-market LSD activities but also over those involving amphetamines, barbiturates, and tranquilizers.

In that year the bureau started training special psychedelic detectives who appropriately enough took their course at the Berkeley campus of the University of California. By 1967 almost two hundred agents staffed special regional bureaus in Atlanta, Baltimore, Boston, Chicago, Dallas, Denver, Kansas City, New York, and Los Angeles. These rookie recruits were also authorized for the first time to carry pistols and to make outright arrests. At the same time, an FDA official admitted that "we do not anticipate that this type of law enforcement will provide all of the answers to drug-abuse control."

The users of heroin and what is termed "heavy drugs" can usually be found on street corners. They congregate in certain areas near the supply that the police can easily stake out. But with LSD the problem is not that simple. As an official of New York City's Narcotics Bureau put it: "What the hell are we supposed to do about LSD? Where do we look? We can't stake out all the colleges and high-rent apartments. And more than that, who is taking the LSD? It could be anybody—people out in Queens as well as the Village crowd—even the pushers who are mostly free-lance. There are no spots, no drops, no nothing. I'm only half kidding but the whole thing would be simpler if the pros moved in completely."

Such bafflement became typical of the agents trying to identify the type of person guilty of violating the anti-LSD laws. Authorities continue to survey known "drops" as the most convenient places to catch those trafficking in acid simply because they have no other leads. Lately, however, police raids have invaded what had been, up until then, the sacred grounds of college campuses. In California, Arizona, and Michigan, state police have used funds from their narcotics departments to pay informers to finger their fellow students involved in drug transactions on campuses as the only sure way of obtaining a conviction.

Despite the work of the agents, a conservative estimate puts the number of persons who use LSD regularly at fifty thousand. Others think an estimate of 150,000 to 250,000 to be more realistic figures. But whatever the disparity in these conjectures, it is generally agreed that the number of persons taking LSD for nonmedical purposes is steadily increasing.

Food and Drug Bureau files analyzing the market show that buyers are generally between the ages of eighteen and thirty, most of them students or dropouts. LSD users, however, are said to include doctors, lawyers, business executives, and theologians; it is no longer strictly an urban phenomenon confined to hippie communities in San Francisco's Haight-Ashbury district or New York's East Village. Of the just under one million bootleg doses of hallucinogens seized by FDA agents in 1967, all geographical areas of the country were represented. In New York City, agents operating out of offices at 201 Varick Street, made 257 arrests and bagged almost 180,000 doses of LSD (more than two and a half million dollars worth). California, the national leader in "acid popping," had close to half-a-million illegal trips aborted by police intervention.

In 1966 the federal government estimates on illegal distribution of LSD put the yearly black-market sale at approximately a million doses, which were sold from seventy-five cents to fifteen dollars per hundred microgram dose. Estimates for 1967 put the figure between five and ten million doses, leaving no doubt that the illegal sale of LSD is on the upswing.

When the restrictions were first laid down, most of the black-market acid came from Europe and Mexico. For a time the Mafia threatened to step in and monopolize the business; Italian pharmaceutical companies—the bane of United States drug firms because they do not recognize drug patents—were rumored to be in cahoots with Mafia smugglers. One major Italian firm was selling the drug for ten thousand dollars a kilogram, which would put the wholesale cost of a 250-microgram trip at two for a penny.

The nature of the market and the small outlay needed to set up in business causes competition to flourish—the main reason for the Mafia's failure to monopolize the acid traffic. The Mafia was further discouraged from appropriating this lucrative field because, unlike the heroin addict, the LSD user is never desperate for the drug. He can take his time shopping around for a good price and he can do without the drug when the supply is down. And even confirmed acidheads don't trip more than once or twice a week.

Regular Mafia distribution outlets were based on their heroin and pill pushers who could be expected to have a bit of trouble infiltrating unnoticed into campus or intellectual circles. The nonaddictive nature of the drug and the invasion of the acid-retailing field by hordes of Mexico-touring amateurs and weekend chemists presented a situation that could not easily be bent to the sway of organized crime. What the Mafia was up against in the early years were, in some cases, young men working their way through college or similar youthful entrepreneurs. A young man or woman could bum around Europe for the summer and return with enough LSD in a pack of cigarettes to pay for the trip and a good share of the coming year's college expenses.

In the manufacturing field, there is no doubt that LSD started its black-market career in the hands of the more adventuresome of the country's budding scientists. As noted previously, the production and sale of acid can be an extremely lucrative business. Using a self-made laboratory, a good organic chemist or chemistry student with the right ingredients can turn out enough LSD to supply half the country. And quite a few entrepreneurs with the know-how took advantage of the opportunity to turn a profit. Their task was made easier by the fact that prior to

1966 one could still legally purchase lysergic acid from such companies as the Sigma Chemical Company in St. Louis for approximately fifty to seventy-five dollars a gram and a good many people were doing exactly that. Once the Food and Drug Administration became aware of the extent of such clandestine operations, it stopped all sales of lysergic acid by chemical suppliers to any unidentified customers.

Earlier, the commissioner of the Food and Drug Administration had asked the chemical suppliers for a list of customers purchasing substances that could be turned into psychedelic drugs. The chemical companies responded to his pleas with less than enthusiasm. A short time later, the FDA took sterner action by outlawing all sales of lysergic acid for use in the manufacture of LSD.

Legal research with LSD, meanwhile, was still being carried on in various centers across the country, but suddenly in 1966 the sole legal producer and distributor of LSD for clinical investigations, Sandoz Pharmaceuticals of Hanover, New Jersey, pulled the drug off the experimental market because of "unforeseen public reactions."

This move led to angry outbursts from researchers using the drug for experimental purposes. Dr. Craig Burrell, medical director of Sandoz's American branch in Hanover, New Jersey, defended his firm's action:

> LSD still has no proven place in medicine. You'll find no one to say the world needs LSD the way it, say, needs penicillin. And in recent years it has become an unmanageable sort of a giant and an amazing user of corporate time. Every time something about LSD gets into the papers, we get dozens and dozens of letters from doctors, asking for the bibliography, and it's already ten inches thick. We've even had people—there were a couple of Harvard students—come to the door, asking for samples.

Federal intervention, however, failed to stop the underground spread of the drug in the same way that Prohibition did little to stop the use of alcohol and the narcotics laws proved inadequate in controlling the use of heroin. In fact, as our campus hippie predicted, the ban appears to have elevated LSD in the popular imagination, surrounding its use with an aura of romantic rebellion against the Establishment forces. Underground intellectuals and hippies were all the while quietly setting up their vacuum pumps and glass beakers to keep campus and bohemia supplied with the prized commodity.

It had been known for some time that a psychedelic trip could be had by chewing on a handful of morning-glory seeds—mainly, "Heavenly Blue" and "Pearly Gates." The underground psychochemical factories discovered that morning-glory seeds were a good source of lysergic compounds. They found that a kilogram of "Heavenly Blue" seeds could yield about twenty-five grams of lysergic acid amide, which gives the underground chemist more than three grams of LSD. "Pearly Gates" morning-glory seeds offered an even better yield because they contain about twice as much lysergic acid.

While the underground chemical factories were churning out LSD for the campus and hippies, the FDA agents had not been sitting still. Their first major success came with the cracking of an LSD ring in Canada in 1963. A New York student and a Toronto actor had been manufacturing the drug on a massive scale and selling it in the United States for five dollars a cube until their apprehension by an undercover FDA agent posing as a buyer.

The FDA was also notified of an LSD scandal in New York City, involving allegations that school and college laboratories were being used for production of the drug. The city's education officials issued denials and refused to allow detectives to invade the chemistry laboratories. In California, not far from Berkeley, where the Food and Drug Administration was training agents, a factory for producing enormous supplies of LSD was uncovered in the attic of a house.

One of the biggest and most recent raids by the federal agents occurred in New York early in 1968 when agents from the New York regional office prevented fifty-four thousand doses of the illegally produced hallucinogens from reaching the city's underground market. An elaborately planned raid on a locked building on Chambers Street, not far from the mayor's office, closed down a potential psychedelic supermarket.

In addition to Drill's *Pharmacology* and numerous other texts on chemistry and drugs, the premises contained an exquisitely equipped laboratory and enough raw material to turn on a good percentage of the city. At five dollars a trip the proprietor stood to gross a quarter-of-a-million dollars on an investment of perhaps ten thousand dollars. The lab had a potential, the bureau agents said, of turning out fifty thousand doses of LSD a day. The agents admit that there must be dozens or hundreds more like them producing LSD on both smaller and larger scales.

A recent investigation by the *New York Post* revealed that there are two kinds of LSD chemists—those who produce acid only for themselves and a few close friends, and those who make acid for wider sale. Among the former, the reporter discovered a doctor and a young Brooklyn chemist, while the latter category included a laboratory technician who moonlighted by making small batches of LSD to be sold on the black market. The reporter also discovered many small acid factories in apartments throughout the city.

According to a recent article in *Newsweek,* the most famous of the alleged underground acid producers is Owsley Stanley. Known as the "Acid King" of the nation's psychedelic community, he is, at thirty-three, surrounded by a mythology as elaborate as that of a regal personage. He is credited with such daring activities as the dispatch of an "Acid Bible" in 1966 to friends jailed in San Francisco for a Civil Rights sit-in. The presoners simply cut up the "Bible," swallowed the marked pieces of Scripture, and were off on their trip.

He is said to have supplied the LSD punch served at the famous "Acid Test" parties in California where hundreds of hippies got "stoned" together and danced to the music of the Grateful Dead, a local acid-rock band.

Hailed as the manufacturer of the best LSD to be had on the hallucinogenic market, Owsley started his career as a youngster with an aptitude for science and stimulants. In the ninth grade he was expelled for "intoxication and bringing intoxicating beverages to school." He is supposed to have supplied good acid out of his laboratory behind a vacant store in Berkeley, according to those who were in a position to sample a lot of it. They praised all his products—the white capsules and the famous blue "Owsley" tabs; and the variety of colors stamped with the figure of Batman and bearing exotic names, such as "Midnight Hours," "White Lightning," and "Monterey Purple." They said that others were producing acid adulterated with "speed" (methedrine), but "Owsley Acid" became a brand they could trust.

In December, 1967, Owsley and four companions were arrested in a San Francisco suburb, where federal authorities at the same time seized more than two hundred grams (almost half a pound) of LSD. This was enough at the standard Owsley dose of 250 micrograms for almost one million tablets that would retail at approximately five million dollars. Also seized were 261 grams of STP, the new supercharged hallucinogen that Owsley is falsely credited with having invented.

Despite such arrests, the battle against its use and distribution continues to be a losing one. Late in 1968, in fact, Attorney General Ramsey Clark stated at a meeting of the National Coordinating Council on Drug Abuse Education and Information: "We can't enforce a law people don't agree with," and went on to concede that laws against marijuana and LSD probably cannot be enforced without broad public approval and cooperation.

Clark informed the council—which is concerned with educating the public to the growing problem of drug use among the young—that any information-education program directed at potential drug users must be based on solid, well-researched fact and not on old-wives' tales. "Young people today are too bright, too quick, too well-educated, and too skeptical."

Attorney General Clark also explained the formation and organization of the Bureau of Narcotics and Dangerous Drugs, a new government agency that had just been set up in the Justice Department. Its duties are to coordinate the activities formerly covered by the Treasury and Health, Education, and Welfare departments whose two enforcing agencies—the Bureau of Narcotics and the Bureau of Drug Abuse Control—were brought together in an attempt to achieve a more efficient enforcement of the drug laws.

Surgeon General William Stewart, head of the United States Public Health Service, speaking at the same meeting, agreed with the Attorney General: "The youth of today," he said, "are extremely sophisticated about drugs and they are also highly selective of the wave lengths they tune in on—the channels of information they select."

It is to be hoped that the selectivity of which Surgeon General Stewart speaks will govern the choice of this extremely important social group, for it now seems likely that not only are their own destinies at stake but that of unborn generations as well. In 1967, more horror stories about LSD were exposed to an already almost hysterical public when the drug came under strong suspect as a possible cause of chromosome damage and birth defects. New research had concentrated on two important areas: (1) the long-range effects of defective chromosomes that might lead to physical or mental abnormalities in the user or in the user's children; and (2) the more immediate potential for defects in the offspring of mothers who had used LSD while pregnant.

The first issue remains unresolved at this moment. The initial report about the use of LSD and possible chromosome damage, published in *Science* Magazine, involved a test-tube experiment during which the drug was injected into human tissue with subsequent damage to cell chromosomes. In a series of additional studies of actual LSD users, the researchers found that the chromosomes of the individual volunteers were damaged. It was impossible, however, from the studies to determine whether or not the chromosome damage was present before the subjects had taken LSD, or had resulted from use of the drug. Accordingly, no real scientific conclusions could be drawn. With the research still incomplete, we cannot take for granted that the appalling possibility is not a real threat.

The studies of the second possible harmful effect of LSD show an even more alarming bent, considering that millions of Americans have used the drug and that infants in the womb are highly susceptible to the effects of any drug—as witness the thalidomide disaster. In another report, also published in *Science* Magazine, it was learned that only one out of five rats injected with LSD early in pregnancy had a normal litter; similar rats that were not dosed all delivered healthy litters. In rats dosed late in pregnancy there was no obvious effect on the offspring.

So far there has been no evidence in human subjects to confirm these disturbing suspicions, but mothers who admitted using LSD during the first three months of pregnancy have delivered normal infants, showing that the drug does not invariably cause congenital defects. There have been, however, reports of malformed children from mothers who did take LSD during pregnancy.

Thus, it would be foolhardy indeed for an expectant mother to knowingly use the drug. She would be gambling with a stake that doesn't even belong to her, the eyesight or the limbs—the very life—of another, and in the broader view, with society at large.

CHAPTER FIFTEEN

TUNING IN: HOW LSD WORKS

Preparing to Leave Ground Control

No two acid trips are alike, for the direction a trip takes depends on the personality of the subject and all the variables in the individual's make-up. The mighty impact of LSD propels the personality bulwark of a lifetime into the background of the psyche. The sweeping transformation affects all the social-value systems—moral and esthetic—and the selective preferences of each of the five senses. That is why it is so difficult—almost impossible—to describe objectively the general effects of the powerful compound.

Like dynamite, LSD must be "handled with care." Even its most ardent champions warn against the casual use prevalent among most acidheads and occasional trippers. Acid tears away the many different masks behind which we all normally hide. Its effects can be especially devastating upon the person whose conditioning has compelled him into so static a code of behavior that he desperately needs a whole battery of such defenses, vanities, and hypocrisies for his everyday survival. Although these are the very people who will benefit most from LSD therapy, they are also the bad trippers. Their ventures into the psychedelic world must embark from just the right set and setting, and be piloted by a master guide of the LSD experience.

Just what do the LSD cognoscenti mean by "set and setting"? According to Timothy Leary, who first defined "set and setting," set refers to the acid user's state of mind before he partakes of

LSD. It includes his previous knowledge of the drug's actions, his expectations and fears about the experience, his personality's effect on the episode to come, and any life-long material that will come into play during the trip.

The environment in which the drug experience takes place is known as the setting. It depends on any physical feature that might influence the occasion—the impression of the room and furniture on the subject if the trip takes place indoors, or the impact of the natural surroundings, if outdoors; the intrusion of music or any other auditory disturbances; the esthetic background and the comfort and security of the subject.

It must be mentioned here that the subject will not be absolutely comfortable and secure if he suffers from a serious physical ailment that might be aggravated by the drug. A complete physical and mental examination of the subject, and a session briefing him in the properties of the drug, should take place at some time in this period of preparation to weed out those tendencies that might so threaten the trip.

Research has indicated that persons afflicted with respiratory problems or cardiac malfunction are poor subjects for the LSD experience because of how their systems might react to the intense emotional impact of the drug. Those with past histories of mental disorder, psychoses, or other related disturbances—including psychological conflicts—are bad risks, too. Even undue anxiety concerning the trip is reason enough to postpone or cancel out the session.

For the most part, only a warm, supportive atmosphere can lead to a therapeutic LSD experience. It was soon discovered that the cold, clinical environment of the first official LSD trips hampered therapy. Actually, early researchers reported that volunteers often refused to renew the experiments. Such experience led many of these first researchers to the conclusion that set and setting were the most important components of an acid trip, although there is a contingent of experts who emphasize the importance of the subject's personality.

Today, those who administer LSD take every precaution to make sure that favorable conditions exist before letting anyone take a "trip." Because unfamiliar settings have occasionally triggered paranoia-like reactions in subjects, this threat, too, is always taken into consideration by acquainting the "tripper" with his surroundings before "getting started." If the session is to take place indoors, the subject is first permitted to examine the room by walking around in it and observing the furniture and the various objects. This makes for a pleasant familiarity with his surroundings, which will contribute to his general feeling of relaxation and security before and during the trip. Another ideal psychedelic setting is an attractive outdoor environment such as a beach, garden, forest, or country retreat.

In addition to the physical surroundings, the setting should include a variety of objects calculated to help the subject enjoy his session. Such accouterments as flowers, stones, seashells, paintings, art reproductions, a collection of records or tapes establish a mood and atmosphere that are additional determinants of the direction the trip might take. The subject should choose these items himself because he is the best judge of what will give him the most pleasure.

During the briefing session, the candidate should be made to understand that the value of his experience will depend in large measure on his willingness to suspend or abandon his ordinary everyday way of looking at things. He should be made to realize that the psychedelic drug will affect him whether he wants it to or not—that is, it is likely that his values and concepts will be completely eradicated when the drug takes hold.

Some candidates, resisting the effects of the drug out of fear that their personalities or their "selves" are being destroyed, are inclined to put up defensive barriers to nullify the drug's action. The subject should be aware that what is being destroyed for the nonce is not his true "self," but the abstract formulation of values and concepts society has imposed upon him. They are, of course, a part of him, but if his reliance on them is so heavy that he panics upon their loss, it is clear that he has never realized the possibilities of his true self. Such a subject is to be urged to confront the experience with complete honesty.

One may draw a parallel with a situation wherein the individual suddenly finds himself in a foreign culture that he must evaluate by its standards and not those of his particular background, if he is to gain an accurate picture of its accomplishments. In a like manner, the acid tripper is plunged into an unknown region where he will recognize images from his own life without, however, the gloss that he or society has placed upon them.

All these possibilities should be laid before the candidate prior to the session. He should be made to understand that the use of marijuana, the amphetamines, and other drugs is not sufficient preparation for an acid trip. A good week of preparation concentrated on the LSD experience is not an undue length of time before the subject embarks on his first LSD trip. Psychologists emphasize that there is no room on the voyage for the irresponsible traveler.

The problem now is "getting started." This, of course, involves every subject's natural resistance to the drug. The proper set and setting already described can now be enhanced by such additional aids as yoga, breathing exercises, a selection of music appropriate to the personality of the subject, a massage, or anything that would put him in a more relaxed frame of mind. The subject may, however, continue to evade the effects of the LSD drug.

Over the years, researchers have observed and noted the many tricks LSD subjects use to avoid involvement in the psychedelic experience. Signs of resistance may progress into actual physical symptoms, such as a trembling due to chill, feelings of nausea and dizziness, acute stomach pains, a restlessness causing the subject to pace back and forth, backaches, and the like. These symptoms are definitely not attributable to LSD but are psychosomatic signs that the subject is fighting the onset of the LSD effects.

Another evasion technique is an insistence on talking continually throughout the session. Words are abstract extensions of structures commonly accepted as real and their persistent evocation tends to restrict the LSD effects. Most of the LSD experience takes place in a nonverbal region of the mind, and deliberate overintellectualization stands in the way of the free flow of the subject's stream of consciousness. In such subjects resistance to the drug is apt to remain high and they are unlikely to make the desired breakthrough.

This is the point at which the trip guide, the second most important influence on an acid session, takes over. Viewpoints differ concerning the best type of guide, but the point on which doctors and researchers concur is that the subject must have implicit trust in his guide. Although Leary claims that professional accreditation of a guide is no guarantee for a good trip, doctors like Houston and Masters suggest strict prerequisites for the proper trip guide. Since the guide is the one who conducts the acid session—leading, assisting, and manipulating the subject, if necessary, over the unfamiliar terrain of his expanded consciousness—he must be a versatile individual. His functions may include that of nursemaid and baby-sitter, priest and troubleshooter, soul mate and sympathetic ear, scullery maid and mother, and any other role the situation may demand. The competent guide never forgets that it is the subject's session and not his. He must be adaptable to any of the eventualities of an acid session; and he must leave his own emotional involvements behind for the eight to ten hours of the session.

The preferred guide is one who has already gone through the LSD experience himself and is capable of preparing the subject emotionally for the session. It is his responsibility to roughly outline what can be expected during the trip and to break down any misconceptions the subject may still have about the experience. In short, he must establish himself as a father figure worthy of respect and trust.

An LSD trip, according to Houston and Masters, will show the subject the manifold aspects of reality—a reality that does not unfold upon a single level or within a single event, but involves a great variety of events on a number of levels. As the experience becomes more profound, the spectrum of sensations and feelings becomes almost infinite.

According to researchers:

> Once the threshold of altered consciousness has been crossed, we are flooded with a kaleidoscopic vision of extended perceptual fields and psychological insights; a visionary torrent of cultures and contacts, myths and symbols, remnants of what may seem to be racial or transpersonal memory—that near-infinity of components that appears to constitute our being . . . It should be one of the chief tasks of the guide . . . to help the subject select out of the wealth among which he finds himself some of the more promising opportunities for heightened insight, awareness and integral understanding that the guide knows to be available in the psychedelic experience.

Not unexpectedly, Masters and Houston adopt a much stricter view on the qualifications and functions of the guide than do people like Leary and Alpert: He should, they insist, be mentally and emotionally stable and possess the capacity to stimulate feelings of security and trust; he should also possess enough savoir faire in his function to manipulate the subject when necessary without appearing to dominate or otherwise interfere unduly with the experience. It is also highly desirable that, along with a good practical knowledge of human psychology, he possess a broad background including a familiarity with history, literature, philosophy, mythology, and religion. Materials from all of these fields, and others, emerge in many of the sessions and the guide must recognize and handle them if he is to be of maximum effectiveness.

A question of controversy has arisen about whether or not the guide should be a user of LSD. The National Institute of Mental Health, the sole distributor of LSD in the United States, once cut off all grants to LSD researchers who had admitted using the drug themselves, regardless of whether they had done so professionally or not. The conservative commission claims that a guide who has participated in a session himself can have neither the proper objectivity nor the ability to manipulate the subject or evaluate the outcome of the session.

Masters and Houston, who have done much experimental research with hundreds of volunteers, emphatically deny the validity of this position. They argue, like Leary, that the guide himself should have been a subject at least once and preferably twice.

> Since the psychedelic experience includes so many elements that are not a part of nondrug state experience, the guide never will be able to understand the subject or communicate with him adequately unless the guide himself has first-hand knowledge of the drug state and its phenomena. This point has become controversial but we see no sound reason why it should be. The argument that the person who has taken psychedelic drugs thereby disqualifies himself as a person able to objectively view and evaluate the experience must strike most seasoned researchers as simply ludicrous. It is also unanswerable, since all who might reply to it on the basis of real knowledge are declared in advance to be unfit to deal with the question. Work done by those who refused to take the drugs does not demonstrate greater objectivity than that of persons who have had the drug experience; and doubtless refusal to experience the psychedelic state is a product, in some cases, of anxiety about the person's ability to cope with that state.

Houston and Masters even see some genuine advantages if the guide takes LSD along with the subject. They do stress, though, that in this case a third person who has not taken the drug should be present during the session. Most researchers agree that the guide's taking anything above a twenty-five microgram dose necessitates the presence of a third person. It is said that a small amount of the drug helps to establish "better rapport between the guide and the subject and also eliminates the possibility of boredom on the part of the guide since the session may take from eight to ten hours with the subject sitting silently and motionless for a good part of that time."

One of the main differences between LSD and other drugs is that the subject on LSD is unable to differentiate hallucinations from reality and is unable to control that differentiation.

The user of marijuana knows that his high is a temporary condition caused by smoking pot, but the person under the influence of LSD is frequently unable to connect his disturbing state of mind to the fact that he has taken a drug. It is at this point that the guide shows his usefulness as a counselor, gently emphasizing to the fearful subject that his hallucinations are the result of nothing other than the LSD he has absorbed in his system.

The candidate, of course, has tried to fix that as strongly as possible in his mind prior to the session as part of the preparation for the trip. He should have acquainted himself to the fullest extent with the basic facts of the psychedelic experience before the session. Nevertheless, the experience might well short-circuit by reason of his attempt to fly or to walk on water. Here again, the guide steps in to provide the subject with a firm perspective, showing in his attitude that he is not treating him in a cavalier manner by "putting him on"—that is, misrepresenting reality during the session.

The delicacy of such rapport is underscored by the fact that the subject's value system is practically nil during the time he is under the influence of the drug, and he will be completely open to any interpretations the guide might impose on his reactions. In a sense, the subject is lost in a strange land and will rely on the guide in the same way as a tourist in a foreign city relies on maps or someone to show him about. In the LSD session, the guide keeps the subject from feeling disoriented and losing control. The feeling of panic at being cast adrift is probably the most disagreeable experience of the trip and is the reason an unguided trip is dangerous and may lead to a state of shock or worse.

Although it is difficult to impose a schedule or any type of structuring upon the psychedelic session, the subject can be bound to certain confines on his trip. He may seemingly veer wildly in his psychic journey, but if the guide "plays it by ear," as much as circumstances allow, he will be able to keep his influence at a minimum and allow the subject to go his own way without any harmful effects. Failing to do so may arouse new feelings of hostility and anxiety in the subject—in this instance, toward the experience.

After set and setting and guide, the third important component of an acid session is dosage. The first thing LSD does is to break down the subject's normal categorical orientation. Although the dosage has some effect on this process, it is not all-important. For someone who knows how to handle the impact of the drug, a small dose may take him exactly where he wants to go. However, someone who inwardly fears the powers of LSD and therefore resists its action may take a massive dose and still be capable of counteracting the drug's effects of personality breakdown. Because of this initial fear of "letting go," researchers suggest that a massive dose be administered to get the subject going, followed by a second, or booster, dose within two or three hours after the first to help break down the threshold of resistance. This, of course, is connected with the set of the subject's mind. If all fear of the drug has been eliminated, and the tripper understands that he must "flow" with the drug rather than fight it, the session will be more successful and dosage will assume a lesser importance.

LSD is the most powerful psychedelic drug known, and it is measured in the smallest unit possible—the microgram, which constitutes a millionth of a gram. About twenty-five to thirty micrograms are enough to have some effect on humans.

Although LSD is usually absorbed in pure form, a number of black-market manufacturers have taken to mixing acid with a number of other drugs, specifically speed, the amphetamine family of drugs. Some specific researchers have found that by mixing LSD with substances such as ritalin, librium, methedrine and the other amphetamines, they have succeeded in obtaining better results.

Scientists have also discovered that certain tranquilizers can be used to end the acid session should the subject lapse into a state of severe anxiety or shock. College students, in fact, frequently use the easily available librium. They have also discovered that by using small amounts of ascorbic acid (vitamins B-3 and C) along with the librium and LSD, they can guarantee a good trip by reducing confusion and anxiety.

For pure LSD, the approximate effects of the drug are as follows:

(1) Twenty-five to seventy-five micrograms have an effect similar to that of marijuana. The general influence of this range is mainly sensual—that is, it alters sensual perception and, like marijuana, it makes the subject more sensitive to auditory and visual stimuli. Consciousness is not perceptibly altered.

(2) One hundred to two hundred and fifty micrograms create altered awareness as well as altered perceptions; analytical and psychological matters preoccupy the subject's consciousness. While the first dosage usually breaks down the subject's sensory perception—causing the physical appearance of things to change and to be re-evaluated—the second dosage usually affects his psychological and sexual make-up. The structures and the masks he has built up over the years suddenly disappear, and he is cast free to ponder on the ultimate reality of things without restraint. The unconscious substrata of his mind often emerge in this state.

(3) Three hundred to six hundred micrograms take the individual to the profound levels of what has been termed the religious or mystical experience. In this state he may feel "a great love for all things in the cosmos" and a "oneness with God."

(4) Six hundred micrograms and over enable the individual to encompass the "cellular structure of biological matter" and "the molecular structure of physical reality."

Perceptions of this kind gave Leary his comprehension of the DNA molecular structure of heredity. It should be pointed out, though, that none of these doses are definitely clear-cut in their effects. An individual may experience all of these states, or perhaps only part of one state during his session, no matter what dose is administered. And there is no such thing as "overdosing" in the sense that taking too much of the drug may prove harmful. Humans have imbibed as much as two thousand micrograms of LSD without any harmful effects. (The lethal dose to humans is as yet unknown.)

There are, of course, many other variables that affect the

dose aside from the subject's psychological make-up. Body weight is one of the determining factors. A person weighing 250 pounds usually requires a larger dose than a person weighing only 150 pounds. Since women usually weigh less, they require only about seventy-five percent of the dose required by men. Experiments carried out with alcoholics in Canada have shown that they require a larger dose, and it has been discovered that heroin addicts require approximately twice the dosage needed to achieve effects similar to those of nonaddicts.

It has been observed that resistance may still remain high in an individual who shows none of the above symptoms. A person sitting quietly, seemingly undergoing the acid experience, may be hung up and unable to make the passage into the realm of psychedelia. Here the subject is on the border line, resisting the effects of the drug and not able to make up his mind whether to let go or to continue to hold off. As stated previously, in some cases this indecision creates fear and even panic. In other cases the subject may simply refrain from going ahead. In such an instance many researchers suggest a booster shot of LSD. This second dose will propel him completely out of his established contexts, making him incapable of maintaining the "self-contact" as he has known it. The Canadian therapists working with alcoholics followed a similar procedure by using very massive doses of the drug to break down the individual's ego defenses.

There are just too many variables to make the prescribed dosage for an individual any more than a rough approximation of what the drug can be expected to do for him during his first trip. Like set and setting and guide, dosage has to be personalized and only experience will establish a subject's needs. As you will see in the next chapter, the effects of the drug—both physical and psychological—depend on the individual, too, and while we can generalize somewhat, they are almost unique in each instance of use.

CHAPTER SIXTEEN

TURNED ON: THE IMPACT OF LSD

Altering Senses and Expanding Consciousness

One ounce of LSD is enough to yield three hundred thousand full doses. Thirty-five pounds of the drug can turn us all on—every man, woman, and child in the United States. The average dose is one hundred micrograms—an amount that cannot be seen without a microscope—and as little as twenty micrograms are sufficient to produce a reaction in an individual.

The drug takes hold in fifteen minutes to one hour and its effects last for approximately eight to ten hours. Its full intensity becomes apparent after one and a half hours. Four hours after taking the drug the effects begin to wane and the LSD subject begins to come down.

It is not known exactly how LSD works on the body during this time. Researchers have discovered, however, that its action is mainly on the diencephalon, or the midbrain. This part of the brain modulates and controls emotional responsivity, consciousness, and dozens of physiological functions from pupil dilation to body temperature.

The pharmacologists were surprised to learn how soon the human body develops a tolerance for the drug. A subject who has taken a dose on three consecutive days shows a complete disappearance of psychic effects on the fourth day, and would have to abstain for from three to four days before another dose of the drug would have any effect on him.

It has been discovered that the body changes occurring during the first hour following LSD ingestion are more psychological than physiological. Such physical symptoms as chills, stomach- or backache, a desire to sleep, trembling, restlessness, a tightening of the muscles, tenseness, drowsiness, and other signs of physical discomfort have all been connected with the body's attempts to ward off the oncoming effects of the drug. Dilation of the pupils, loss of appetite, and temperature changes in the body are some of the few observable effects. Oddly enough, some individuals who have taken repeated doses of the drug manifest no initial physical symptoms at all.

The first noticeable effects of LSD are primarily on the five senses: sight, hearing, touch, smell, and taste. Colors seem more vivid and luminous; hearing becomes more acute; the sense of touch is intensified. These are not actual physical exaggerations of the sensory apparatus, but a breakdown of the categorizations that make such sensory perceptions commonplace.

A child sees his first bright red ball, tastes his first piece of chocolate, smells his first flower, touches his first piece of velvet, and hears his first few notes of music in a manner not unlike that of the individual under LSD. As the child grows into man, experience jades his perceptual apparatus; the new and unexpected become the commonplace and routine, fading into the peripheral consciousness where it lies half-buried. Under LSD these primary sensations are unusual and moving once again.

This capacity to bring back the impact of the new results from isolation of the sensory mechanism from all related meaning. Perception under LSD is no longer subservient to meaning and the sensations become just that. A blaring police siren is not associated with emergency or danger, but is a sound—to be appreciated for its own sake. So it is with all objects and sensations.

One of the unique properties of the drug is that it excludes random distractions from the immediate perception and permits total concentration. The object focused upon assumes a profound significance. The subject and the object seem to merge, and there appears to be a selfless relationship in the perception. The other senses are similarly affected. The subject listening to music may become completely absorbed in the experience; texture and shape yield their qualities in the most profound manner to the sense of touch; the absolute essence of any scent is penetrated by the olfactory senses. Time is drastically altered—it speeds up, slows down, reverses, and sometimes disappears completely. A most common effect is a retardation in which centuries seem to go by, and the second hand on the watch appears to stand still.

Often, when the subject leans back and closes his eyes, he can visualize a most colorful and striking array of geometric patterns—a veritable kaleidoscope of images that range from liquid swirls to wallpaper-type designs. Another perceptive alteration appears in the seeming movement of static objects: Walls give the impression of undulating, as if they were composed of rubber; faces appear distorted, as if they are being observed through a wide-angle lens; and objects such as sofas and flowers seem to breathe.

One of the pleasant effects of the drug is synthesia—a cross-over of sensations in which the subject "tastes" music and "hears" colors. Rhythmic sounds seem to control and conduct a color symphony that can be viewed from behind closed eyes.

LSD affects space to a lesser degree. However, there is some distortion and certainly a person under the influence of LSD should not attempt to drive an automobile. The problems that arise during this sensory level involve unpleasant fantasies of a physical nature. The subject may become so affected by the increased psychedelic body sensitivity that he may develop delusions that he is bleeding to death, suffering from a wound in one of his organs, or is in the throes of some horrible disease. These are, however, hallucinations, and the guide should be able to divert the subject.

In this state there is also a breakdown of the normal structures of time and relationships; if the subject attempts to cling to the old predrug-state frame of reference, he may be in for some tortuous moments. Unless he goes along with the psychedelic tide, he will be overcome by anxiety and confusion and may become even more persistent in his efforts to maintain his normal categorical orienttation.

The guide should try to lead him away from this possible hang-up by showing him the power of his expanded sensory consciousness. The guide should point out, for instance, that the subject can turn water into wine simply by thinking it so, and may then hand him a glass of water to reinforce the suggestion; the subject's taste buds will then tell him that the water is wine. This simple ploy should help the subject by drawing his attention to his heightened perception of color and the forms of well-known objects. Examining a common object, the subject will be overwhelmed by a sense of wonder and over the complexity of the most simple items. He will then go on to test his sensory stimuli on paintings, music, or anything else that is not likely to result in personal psychological difficulties, for it is desirable that he first accustom himself thoroughly to the unfamiliar altered consciousness induced by LSD.

After a few hours in this sensory stage, it will be easier for the subject to pass into what Houston and Masters describe as the recollective-analytic stage.

At this new level, the changes induced in the thought processes and the effect of the drug on what Western man calls "the self" are, perhaps, the most dramatic of all its many manifestations. Boundaries are wiped away; the self is no longer separated from the external world. Psychological defenses—those barriers that we put up to defend the integrity of the personality—are broached, and a great amount of repressed material floods the conscious mind.

The emergence of material usually stored in the subconscious may bring on a crisis when the individual is faced with the decision to surrender or hold on to his ego controls. The effects of LSD can be overcome by those who fear the loss of self-identity, although a great deal of anxiety is engendered during an attempt at such resistance. Once these defenses are overcome, however, a covey of personal memories from the deep recesses of the subject's mind will come into focus.

Here again, anxiety may develop, depending on whether these memories are painful or joyous, ugly or beautiful, ludicrous or worthwhile. The subject will find himself observing this material directly and will react accordingly, with feelings of guilt, pride, pleasure, or other emotive behavior.

The social and cultural storehouse contained in the superego also tends to dissolve, suppressing the role of the conscience and opening up doors to past events hitherto buried in oblivion. Under LSD, the individual's social- and ethical-value system does not hinder him from examining the most embarrassing images of his past life. Contrary to the belief held by a few drug authorities that this disinhibition of the conscience parallels the effects of alcohol, the LSD trip seldom includes the kind of acting-out behavior, including sexual, that frequently occurs during inebriation. While the ethical reins are undoubtedly slackened, there is not a total loss of behavior controls.

At the same time, a less dogmatic attitude and a new and greater tolerance for others' viewpoints may develop. This new outlook sometimes lasts for a time following the acid session and may lessen anxiety, if the individual comes to abandon what may have been a burdensome value system and adopt a more flexible and less-constricting one.

This ability of the individual to examine memories, unburdened by feeling of guilt or anxiety, often leads him to believe that at last he is seeing himself as he really is. So astonishing will be this new insight that he may be absolutely overwhelmed, and in his excitement, laugh and cry at the same time. For many, the discoveries mean new truth and wisdom; for a lesser number, they bring about major personality transformation.

The process—highly complex, subtle, and elusive—is very difficult to describe. To an individual under LSD, even a single thought may branch out into a vast hierarchy of related subthoughts, all connected and ramified into a shifting and interconnected pattern. To do more than contemplate this composition is futile and translation into words captures only fragments.

It is this association of ideas riding on the flood of thought that often produces the strongest emotional impact. Thinking and feeling become hardly separable as powerful feelings are joined to thought.

The symbolic level, which Houston and Masters place as the third stage, is a much more intense and less-cerebral stage than the preceding one and may result in a profound self-realization as well as a high degree of selftransformation. At this symbolic level, the hallucinations assume major importance because the individual may begin to participate in an imaginary episode and to react in fear or pain or joy or hate. He may physically act out various scenes in a drama that he believes is taking place at that very moment.

The fourth or integral level has been described variously as a state of union with God, a mystical or religious experience, an illumination similar to Zen Satori, and a sense of complete psychological integration. Houston and Masters explain this level as the one in which "ideation, images, body sensation and emotion are fused in what is felt as an absolutely purposive process culminating in a sense of total understanding, self-transformation, religious enlightenment, and possibly mystical union. The subject here experiences what he regards as a confrontation with the ground of Being, God, Mysterium, Noumen, Essence, or Fundamental Reality."

There is no hangover after the effects of the drug have worn off. Once the subject has come down, he will find himself restored to normal reality. Unlike the hazy flux of the dream sequence, he will remember in detail the experiences of his LSD session.

It is manifestly clear that the dangers and obstacles encountered on an acid trip make it an extremely hazardous experience for the unguided and ill-prepared person. Responsible advocates of the drug have suggested establishing clinics to which the prospective tripper might turn. Many of the youngsters taking the drug do so only to "groove" on the psychedelic hallucinations that accompany it without realizing that the hallucinatory level is elementary and can easily spin out of control with serious results. The volunteer, psychologists warn, should be sufficiently motivated to want the trip for the personal benefits he will derive from it. The clinical setting, including proper medical supervision, is necessary to guide a journey that otherwise might well end up in a house of horrors.

CHAPTER SEVENTEEN

FLYING HIGH: THE MIND UNSHACKLED

The Treasure Trove of the Psyche

It would appear that LSD is a ticket to a wondrous time machine that transports the tripper on a whirlwind tour of mankind's ancestral past. Timothy Leary's LSD experience gave him a glimpse of "God's handiwork in the genetic code imprinted on man's cellular structures." Others have come back aglow with the remembrance of bacchic rites, high masses in medieval cathedrals, offerings to Mayan gods, Hindu temple rites—all the immensely rich life and culture that preceded ours.

The itineraries of many such journeys have been observed by medical authorities and, in the opinion of the authors, are the only accounts that can be admitted into the records as real evidence; the more casual trippers interviewed by the authors, and other researchers in the field, concentrated on the hallucinatory aspects.

The mystifying and often frightening landscape that the LSD subject encounters on his journey inward is staked with many milestones that mark the way a psychotherapist can help him to better health. LSD stimulates an easy recall of events long buried in a patient's subconscious, and striking insights into his own nature and the real world around him. He and a therapist can thus move much faster and far more comfortably toward resolution of even the most paralyzing problem.

Let us here examine the histories of a number of subjects who have undertaken piloted LSD trips in their search for mental health. The experiences recounted are from the dossiers of a wide variety of subjects, ranging in interests and life patterns from housewives to LSD cultists.

Our first subject, Mr. A., is a twenty-nine-year-old junior executive in a middle-sized advertising firm in New York. His Greek-Orthodox parents worked hard to send him through a university, where he combined an English literature major with an intensive study of Arabic. Of small and slender stature, he was always a loner in an athletically oriented high school where he "always felt I didn't fit in."

The central image of his boyhood is a dingy booth in the rear of his father's restaurant where he spent his time, devouring Greek, Scandinavian, and Chinese legends. Although he married a woman whom he insists he loves, he feels that it was arranged by his parents, who had introduced him to her at a barbecue in the backyard of their home.

He was initiated into the rites of LSD through an account executive at the agency who had turned on several times previously and guided a number of persons on the trip. The setting was an apartment on the upper East Side, described by Mr. A. as modern and filled with bric-a-brac and artifacts from his friend's travels:

> We were sitting in B.'s living room, idly talking, when he pulled out a small morocco pouch. He held up a tiny ball of silver foil, which he said contained five hundred micrograms of LSD in two sugar cubes. We swallowed the granular substance.
>
> Nothing happened for about half an hour. I had gotten up a few times to look at a few things in the room and frankly I didn't expect much to happen. Then, suddenly, my body began to tingle. It seemed as if all the pores opened up, like flowers drinking in the colors and substances of the objects around me. The color green was quite delicious; yellow had a tart, bitter-sweet taste that I didn't find disagreeable. The only color I couldn't stomach was a kind of azure blue, which tasted very metallic and left my palate dry. I found red to be very heady and cautioned myself not to "drink" too much of it.
>
> At that time, B. asked me what it felt like to live in an aquarium, and I could see myself swim inside the room, bubbles rising from my mouth. It struck me as quite funny, thinking how I'd appear to the outside world. I thought of myself as an exotic fish with a quick-flashing tail and luminescent body. My

wife appeared behind the glass walls and her body was distorted as if it were reflected in a laughing mirror. Her hand appeared over the top like a large bird and swooped down into the water. But I darted away and each one of her efforts to catch me failed.

For awhile, I hugged the sandy bottom, working a mist of fine dust off the sand with the flashing of my tail. I then entered a large swaying fern that immediately parted its leaves to reveal a beautiful interior of sparkling floors and marble walls, a marvelous sea palace. It was very still; nothing moved and the pumping of my gills made the walls seem to sway slightly.

Suddenly a voice boomed out, commanding me to halt. Straining my eyes, I could see where the voice came from: It belonged to Neptune himself, sitting on a throne of kelp and coral in a robe of resplendent seaweed. He held a golden trident in one hand and a large book in the other. I couldn't refrain from laughing. The book, I discovered, was *The Compleat Angler* by Isaac Walton, which I'd read for an English course in the university. The laughter had aroused Neptune from his regal pose. Three times he brought down the butt end of his trident on the floor, which then opened and tumbled me through a mist of swirling darkness. I remember being quite terrified at the time, but also overcome by curiosity to see where my fall was taking me. As I descended into these mysterious regions, I went through the complete evolutionary cycle. My gills changed to tiny lungs; I sprouted a tail and became a quick, nervous reptile, flicking my tongue at mayflies. Then my legs became longer until finally I could walk erect and swing from tree branches. By the time I got back to earth, I was a fully developed human, alone in an immense cavern where stalagmites and stalactites cluttered my vision. Behind them I could hear the moanings of drowned sailors, the creaking of a half-buried hull of a Spanish galleon. I was overcome by emotion at the thought of these lost people come to rest at some unknown patch of sea bottom in ages past.

All of this seemed to be a physical extension of myself. Somehow I had seen these sailors, this galleon and I had voyaged on feeble ships over uncharted seas. My thoughts were interrupted by an old man covered with barnacles and lichen who announced he was my guide. He carried a walking stick entwined by a sea snake. His steps were sure and he led me to a mossy courtyard where Nereids, goddesses of the sea, performed a magnificent dance that held me spellbound. Then I saw something quite terrifying—the severed head of Medusa floating with streaming, blood-clotted hair above me. A lovely figure appeared, half-snake and half-woman. The guide whispered to me to stay hidden behind a huge shell, for the beautiful figure was known to eat men raw by tearing the flesh from their bodies with coil-like hands.

At that time I must have been very scared because I noticed B. standing over me with a look of concern on his face. He asked if I was all right and I remember saying, "I'm a chicken of the sea," and giggling. I noticed I had the telepathic ability to sense his thoughts, anticipating his every word and move. I thought of the air being vibrant with millions of thought waves silently criss-crossing one another without ever touching. It seemed to me evocative of the human condition—all those people in hundreds of countries and cities not knowing what the other person is thinking. I felt grateful to LSD for giving me a glimpse into the nature of the thought process.

At that time, I told B. to take off his mask. He admitted to having worn a mask all his life, not one but thousands. He said he carried them in multiple layers that he could remove one at a time as the day progressed. He then got up to play a record and instantly the room was filled with a tremendous cascade of sounds. The record was Vivaldi's *Four Seasons* and, although I had enjoyed it many times before, I had never "penetrated" it as much as I did then. The baroque trills had a stately grace, a tone of ascetic leisure that made me wish I had been born in another age. I didn't associate the music with the trite fact of a black disk mechanically spinning on a turntable. That thought depressed me. Instead, I felt the music emanating from many different sources—a desk lamp piping like an oboe, the venetian blinds being plucked like a lute by unseen fingers, a vase trumpeting a solo, a cigarette case on the table clapping its lid like a timpanum. I also thought how trivial and absurd the things were that tied me to my conventional existence. I had such tremendous powers and such great insight into the nature of things that I was saddened at the thought of how I wasted my best energies on a stupid round of daily activities.

I felt that I must have done something awfully evil to be tantalized by the visions I saw without being able to make them permanently mine. It was a punishment, perhaps, for having given up the bright dreams of my youth and exchanged them for a relatively secure and comfortable life without too many problems. I felt myself hemmed in by obstructions, none of which were of my own making but imposed upon me as obligations by society, laws, parents, wife, my job. But there was nothing I could do about it. I felt infinitesimally small against the universe, and unable to influence Providence, stars, or moon—whatever it was I felt was guiding my life.

Mr. A.'s trip left him depressed, but on later reflection he found the whole experience exhilarating for having given him insights into his psyche and the nature of existence that he hadn't thought himself capable of achieving. The experience remained uppermost in his mind for more than a week, interfering somewhat with his work. After that, he found himself more at ease with his environment and embarked on an ambitious reading project into mystical and historical works.

The following LSD experience was described by Mrs. R., a twenty-five-year-old West Coast librarian married to a commercial-airline pilot. During her husband's frequent absences she had engaged in an affair with an art student at the local university; he turned her on. Her marriage was not a happy one on her part. She said her husband was "a good man but a bore." She had been married for four years and had started drinking to combat her increasingly frequent periods of depression. Although she enjoyed her extracurricular affair she felt guilty about it and had thought of terminating it.

The setting of the trip was a national park on the Pacific Coast where she had driven with her lover. When they got to a lonely spot on a hill, they parked the car and wandered down to a sheltered grove by a small stream. Since this was her first psychedelic experience, her companion had suggested that he would refrain from taking the drug to be able to guide her:

> I first noticed the effects of the drug when I opened my compact and caught a glimpse of myself in the small mirror. Staring back at me was an old, wizened face mottled with warts and whiskers. The eyes were sunk deep in the sockcts, the mouth was puckered like the ring of an orange peel, and the skin was blotched by a dull brown color. "Would I look like this when I grew old?" I asked myself. I had once seen a film where a beautiful young girl had been instantly transformed into a wrinkled old hag. That scene immediately came back to my mind and, although I realized that the image I saw was the effect of the drug, I couldn't help feeling depressed at the thought of aging.
>
> Fortunately, at that time, D. asked me what I saw in the

mirror. I told him, and he suggested I hold up the mirror over my shoulder and watch the scudding clouds. Caught in the small frame, it seemed as if I was examining the slowly elongating substance of some form of microscopic life. It appeared to be caught up in a painful, silent agony. I then saw it as a cell groping for union with another to start the mute beginnings of life. Thus I came into existence, I thought: gray tufts of sperm floating aimlessly toward an unforeseen union with ovaries dropping like dew in a golden uterine mist.

My body at the time actually felt weightless. I could feel the ego sense leaving me as I grew lighter and lighter. It was as if I was molting my old skin and receiving a new one of light, shiny texture.

I noticed that. D. had taken off his shirt and was watching me with his hands propped under his head. He immediately struck me as a beautiful young man, although, in reality, he had an interesting, but not handsome face as understood in conventional terms. "You're divine," I told him. He held a flower in his mouth on which he seemed to be playing a seductive tune. I imagined him as a young Greek god frolicking through the woodlands, piping his merry tune. Wood nymphs, lake spirits, elfin gods, and all the animal life of the forest gamboled after him over hills, dales, and streams. I became a white dove turning slow cartwheels in the sky, watching the tiny figures recede into groves and emerge again on a luscious field. It was one of the most beautiful things I've ever seen. In the open meadow, he lay down gazing at the clouds as the sun waxed his limbs. His band of followers had disappeared and a shower of rose petals fell from a magnificent rainbow, flecking his body with tiny flakes of all different colors.

I felt as if he were unaware of my presence and I thought I would really surprise him by appearing out of a clump of bushes like a tree spirit. I got up and, for a few minutes, retired behind a nearby tree where I took off my clothes. While walking, the hill seemed to bounce, rippling like waves with the trees bobbing like the masts of a fleet of wooden schooners. I had never felt as close to nature before, and I realized that I might have been some passive wildflower in a previous existence. With each article of clothing I peeled off, my closeness to the environment seemed to increase. It was as if all of nature silently expressed its approval of my desire to present myself in my natural state.

When I was finally nude, I was overcome by a warmth and sense of comfort that I've never experienced before or since. The pile of clothes on the grass seemed like an obscene article. My brassiere with its two padded cups struck me as being totally ludicrous. The short skirt and limp stockings bore no relation to the human form.

When I returned, D. had also stripped off his clothes. Against the luscious background, parts of his body were unnaturally white. Lying down, we looked for a while at the sky and the swaying treetops, which seemed to huddle in a protective circle around us.

D. took my hand and put it on his chest. It felt strange to feel the hair brush against my skin. At the same time I saw his body not as a whole, but as a multiple of millions of cells, each contributing its bit like the symphony of a harmonious piece of music. When I touched a part of his body it came to life as if my fingers were a magic wand. I noticed his erection. Actually I had watched it swell, like a snake uncoiling itself. I had never really looked at a penis before, finding it somehow gross and somewhat pathetic. Now, for the first time, I really examined it and was stupefied at its power and complexity.

I became aware of the tremendous difference between male and female. The full nature of the sex act, which I'd never really thought about, suddenly became clear to my mind. I was thrilled to find how wondrously it had been arranged—the lock and the key and the mysterious juices that lubricated them. D. was stroking my breasts now. I'm usually not erogenous there, but this time, the slightest pressure multiplied into a vortex of sensation that sent spasms of pleasure into every part of my body. We touched each other with never more than the fingertips but the actual tactile sensations felt as if we were in contact all over.

We lay there exploring each other for a long time until I was seized by a frightening vision. Just as we were at the height of our passion and D. made ready to consummate the act, I saw his penis break off from the crotch and drop, lifeless, to the ground. The sun had disappeared and suddenly the knoll was alive with menacing shadows. I was afraid to speak of what I'd just seen and I grew even more terrified when I thought I could feel my vulva dry up and fill with dust.

D. told me later that I had turned around and curled up in the fetal position. With my eyes closed I saw a figure rise in the sky and address me in thundering tones. It was an awesome appearance—the devil, perhaps. What it said terrified me so much I lay absolutely frozen, unable to move. I was asked to sacrifice D. on a small altar constructed from twigs to pay for my sins. According to D., I was in a frightful state, whimpering and crying words he couldn't understand. I then heard a rumble as if the earth were splitting and both of us were carried away on an immense floodtide where we floated for years until the waters receded.

The entire episode probably didn't take more than minutes and, as the flood subsided, the earth turned once again beautiful and fresh. I heard Debussy's *Afternoon of a Faun* playing softly through the foliage. Around me, the hill took on deep hues like a Tintoretto or Rubens painting while the sun slowly sank with an expression of pain on its face. A whole succession of what appeared to me Indian gods then marched by in single file—Shiva, Kali, the eight-armed Yoga, and the profoundly peaceful face of Buddha. The threat to D. had been averted and we made love to each other for what must have been hours. It was the most satisfying experience of my life. I would advocate the use of LSD for sex purposes without hesitation if it weren't for the unknowable terrifying sensations that may accompany it. It saddened me to think that such profundity of emotion and feeling needed the catalyst of drugs to be activated.

The next case history concerns a thirty-two-year-old Negro musician who claims to have kicked a long-standing heroin addiction with the use of LSD. Mr. X. grew up in South Carolina, studied music and attended college for a time in New York City. He has been making his living as a musician since the age of seventeen. He was married for a few years, "but 'horse' [heroin] ruined that." He turns on with LSD frequently, asserting that the drug affords him dramatic insights into his ancestral past.

The historical roots of his race had been symbolically revealed to him in one of his most memorable experiences. Its most rewarding aspect had been a renewed pride in and consciousness of his Negro past, as well as a movement beyond his individual self to a more profound understanding of his own nature. His music, he says, has benefited from the experience. His most exciting trip took place some time ago at the apartment of a friend—a Negro nationalist who has assumed an African name and wears traditional Yoruba dress:

I had been tripping for a while . . . letting a stream of ideas flow freely without any direction. Then . . . my friend . . . Ombonwe . . . whom I told you about . . . showed me a picture of two Sara dancers from the Republic of Chad. The two figures had been frozen into a graceful rhythmic posture that held a tremendously explosive force. They were wearing beaded loin cloths and bracelets. When I closed my eyes . . . they came alive to the music of drums beating out a staccato rhythm. As the dance grew more frenzied, the music became more insistent and to my surprise I recognized many of the "riffs" I'd played without being aware of their origin.

Soon more people appeared, clapping their hands and shaking their bodies in convulsive movements. The startling thing was that the background against which these dances took place changed constantly. At first, it had been a jungle village with thatched huts and a variety of domestic animals. At that time, something happened that I still can't explain and don't entirely believe. According to Ombonwe, I was uttering certain words that he identified as belonging to the Fon language, spoken in Dahomey, West Africa. I had never heard a word of African before, let alone this obscure language. Subsequent LSD experiences, though, following up on much of what I'd hallucinated previously, failed to bring back this extraordinary phenomenon.

The background suddenly changed and the dancers, now wearing soiled Ironboy overalls, were on a plantation levee. From there, the scene transferred to a West Indian island where the dancers engaged in an act of homage to a king and queen wearing bright red clothes and sandals. A small procession of people brought sacrificial gifts, after which a new dance began in a circle around the king and queen. The air was filled with strange voodoo cries, and magic chants that whipped the dancers into a greater and greater frenzy. At the height of the excitement a number of them fell into a trance and I grew afraid of being discovered by a couple of huge bodyguards with the royal couple. However, the music was irresistible and I couldn't help being caught up in it, tapping my feet and uttering the incantations.

When they found me, I was hauled before the king and queen who turned out to be the high priest and priestess of the proceedings. The priest drew a circle and placed me in the middle of it. I was led to an altar where I was forced to eat a mushroom and take an oath that I would not reveal anything about what I'd seen. The drumming then mounted into a crescendo. The dancers tore off their clothes and surrendered themselves completely to the rhythm. A large snake was brought and tossed onto the grass where it lay writhing. The priest appeared with a rooster which he swung violently around by its legs. The dancers were now completely transported, biting their flesh and smearing their faces with the blood from a number of slaughtered roosters.

I managed to break away and wandered through the forest for

many days. At one point, I sank into a pool of quicksand from which I was rescued by a wise old man who refused to talk and disappeared immediately thereafter. I stumbled blindly on, my vision obscured by swirling mists. This seemed to have gone on for a long time until I came to a seashore where I was forcibly captured and put on a boat. I voyaged for what again appeared to be a long time . . . At that point Ombonwe suggested we get some fresh air on the balcony. I gradually came down, although the experience was forever etched into my mind. I had discovered an unknown part of my previous existence and since then have become extremely interested in Negro history. . . .

The previous accounts show the rich imagery and hallucinations that may accompany the properly supervised LSD trip. According to psychologists, the individual's dramatic involvement serves to release a stream of symbolic visions that bear an uncanny relationship not only to his own past but to his ancestral history as well. The psychedelic experience at its best embodies a mythic substantiation of the universe that is frequently overpowering in its revelations. It is a world of myth and ritual, a never-never land of infinite grace and goodness, or a terrifying landscape of diabolic proportions.

The three sample cases were deliberately chosen from highly intelligent and articulate subjects, for it is not surprising that the person who has experienced the rapid kaleidoscopic flow of images, hallucinations, visions, insights, and ideas of another world finds it difficult to verbalize. The average tripper, as a matter of fact, is usually left speechless, even after the effects have vanished.

In some instances, transformations are far-reaching and may decisively alter the individual's thinking on a number of relevant levels. Personality transformations such as Mr. A. and Mr. X. describe, however, are not always of long duration.

Young people and hippies who use LSD are prone to sing its praises for personality transformations they claim are effected by the drug. But it is exactly against such cavalier attitudes that medical authorities direct their strongest warnings. Occasionally an unguided user of acid may derive similar beneficial results from his trip. But all too frequently he "flips out" and the aftereffects of the psychedelic experience reinforce a paranoia that transforms his personality in ways that are far from desirable. In hippie jargon, "he has blown his mind"—a mental state that may be of shorter or longer duration but that, in the meantime, often leaves the individual incapable or unwilling to carry on with the normal routines of life.

CHAPTER EIGHTEEN

ACID THERAPY: LSD AND MENTAL HEALTH

Neurosis, Psychosis, and Alcoholism

The study of the mind is, indeed, difficult. Man cannot stand apart from its scientific exploration in the manner of the physicist or chemist and his formulae or compounds. Efforts to gather information about the human psyche are further handicapped in that experiments with animals are severely limited by a lack of communication.

As a result, the twin sciences of psychology and psychiatry suffer from the same dual-headed conflict as prescientific medicine. At one extreme stand the strictly objective observations of the behaviorists, which tend to be simplistic and meaningless in the overall view of the problem, while the other end of the spectrum is cluttered with an elaborate tangle of theories—obscure, esoteric, and sometimes, misleading.

This split has kept the field in turmoil from the beginning. The behaviorists condemn the elaborate theories of their contemporaries; they, in turn, are opposed by those who call the concepts of the behaviorist method both limited and useless.

The questions surrounding LSD have added even more to this polarity in viewpoints. The medical establishment tends to favor the viewpoint of the behaviorists. While they explored the strictly medical uses of the new compound, others in the field were taking careful note of the changes in perception and mental activity caused by the drug. Reports were heard of use of the drug for a memorable experience rather than as a therapeutic tool, and a second group grew up around those who were interested in the mystical and spiritual values of LSD.

The medical establishment was, of course, out to limit the drug to researchers who would evaluate its properties as a useful weapon against mental disorders. Behind closed doors, they experimented and kept the drug under wraps for twenty years, but it was inevitable that word would leak out about its dramatic range of mind-altering properties—pleasurable shortcuts to the transcendental and mystical experience. LSD came to be known as a means of obtaining a new and exciting experience, with the result that it attracted not only the serious but also the thrill seekers, the bored, and the unstable.

It is a new social problem that has spread a wave of concern across the United States that continues to grow. Some say the drug disorganizes and disrupts mental activity; others contend that LSD organizes and integrates the mind.

Those involved in early LSD physiological and psychological research hold opinions both pro and con as to its possible value. In the beginning the spiritual-mystical group was not so obvious in its orientation, but as the consciousness-expanding possibilities of LSD became clearer, these two groups split over the medical researchers' expressed disinterest in the drug's transcendental aspects. Of course, the medical-research group was traditionally exempted from entering this field, which was held in some disrepute by the scientific establishment.

In the early 1950's, chemical therapy of mental illness was in its infancy, although medical circles held out great hope for the discovery of compounds that they could apply to a number of these ills of mankind. The opinion at the time was optimistic, chemistry would untangle a good many of the psychiatric problems that had long defied solution. Stocks in pharmaceutical companies round the world soared as they flooded the market with dozens of psychic drugs. The medical profession greeted those new pharmaceuticals with great excitement. Mood elevation and peace of mind could be purchased for the price of a small vial of pills. The popular tranquilizer Miltown and a great variety of pep and sleeping pills were to usher in the new age of psychochemicals.

The same people who condemned the rising popularity of morning-glory seeds, marijuana, and LSD among youngsters were those who were ceaselessly swallowing tranquilizers, popping "bennies," and downing sleeping pills. Apart from this, it soon became obvious that there were more serious benefits to be gained from the pharmaceutical revolution than the relief of minor anxieties and ailments. The first to feel the benefits of this thinking were the overcrowded mental wards, which were able to release many of their patients from straitjackets, padded cells, and chains, and return a good number of them to society after various forms of chemical treatments.

This road to chemical Nirvana was almost blocked in 1962 by the thalidomide scandal. Developed as a mild sedative, thalidomide was found beneficent in calming worried pregnant woman. Unfortunately, it also created some highly undesirable side effects. The appearance in newborns of flippers instead of hands and other tragic deformities deadened enthusiasm over the newly developed pharmaceuticals. The phenomenal sales of chemicals bearing seductive names for minor worries and tensions took a sudden nose dive and the percentage of Americans seeking relief in a pill decreased considerably. There still remained a large enough demand, however, to make such drugs a gold mine for the pharmaceutical companies.

This was the background against which LSD came of age. Early biological research focused on that compound with the hope that it would disentangle the coils of schizophrenia. In the fifties, when Sandoz Laboratories were shipping thousands of samples of LSD to researchers around the country, psychiatrists testing the substance believed that their neurotic patients were finally getting a radically new orientation that might prove to be of immense value in unlocking the subconscious. After these initial favorable reports, Sandoz started preparations to market the drug (even giving it one of those acronyms favored by pharmaceutical companies—Delysid).

Having administered the drug to more than one hundred volunteers, Dr. Max Rinkel, a psychiatrist attached to the Massachusetts Mental Health Center in Boston, sent back reports confirming the European investigations. He was especially struck by the similarity of the drug's effects on normal volunteers to the behavioral symptoms of schizophrenics—the sensation of separating into two distinct personalities, one observing the other; the distortion of time and space; the hallucinations and illusions; and the scattering of rational thoughts and emotions. This raised hopes among the medical experimenters that they were on the way to creating an imitation psychosis in a normal volunteer—a chemical breakthrough that might, in turn, lead to the discovery of another compound capable of counteracting the effects of LSD. An agent of this nature might then be used in the treatment of schizophrenia with a reasonable expectation of success.

The simulation of the actual symptoms of a disease is a prime concern of medical researchers, and LSD was subsequently hailed as a psychotomimetic—a chemical that elicits a psychosis. If a chemical cause of schizophrenia is ever conclusively uncovered, one logical approach to its treatment would be to manufacture an agent capable of producing cross tolerance to it.

The first controversies arising around LSD centered on the question of whether or not it produced a true schizophrenic state or toxic delirium. If LSD caused only a confused delirium, its value and interest to the medical establishment would be minor. But during the first decade of research with the new compound the prevailing belief was that the drug did indeed produce a psychosis. Then scientists began reporting that, despite the parallel to madness, actually something different from an actual psychosis was being induced.

Eventually, a compromise conclusion was reached in which the researchers agreed that LSD did neither exactly mimic schizophrenia nor parallel closely the disorienting delirium. LSD's application as a therapeutic tool was not abandoned, however, since there was enough evidence to substantiate its apparent successful use in a number of other clinical situations. Although it did not prove to be the long-sought-for chemical key to schizophrenia, the drug is known to be effective in treatment of some types of schizophrenia, especially those that afflict children.

In those early years of experiments with LSD therapy, not one instance was recorded that could in any way be interpreted as proof that the drug is harmful. Its use in the treatment of various forms of mental illness was not altogether successful, but nonetheless one of the early reports stated conclusively that LSD does "offer a means for readily gaining access to the chronically withdrawn patients. It may also serve as a new tool for shortening psychotherapy."

There are two schools of thought concerning the use of LSD as a therapeutic tool in the treatment of psychosis. One would restrict the drug to the hands of the therapist for the sole purpose of gaining an insight into the world of schizophrenia; the other seeks to use LSD as a psychochemical in direct application to the patient. The sharp differences between the effects produced by LSD and those observed in the behavior of schizophrenics were recently summarized in a report at New York University:

> The spectacular visual illusory phenomena and perceptual distortions induced by the hallucinogenic compounds is not typical of schizophrenia. However, the de-personalization which some non-psychotic subjects display under the influence of higher doses of these drugs is strikingly similar to what may be seen in acute schizophrenic reactions.

Dr. Humphry Osmond, Director of the Bureau of Research in Neurology and Psychiatry at Princeton, New Jersey, and Dr. Abram Hoffer, a Canadian psychiatrist, believe that LSD may yet provide the key to a cure of schizophrenia. Basing their research on Freud's observation that mental illness may be caused by a chemical imbalance in the body, Drs. Osmond and Hoffer developed a similar theory and were among the first to see the similarities between the LSD effects and schizophrenia. Their findings, however, have largely fallen on deaf ears; LSD as a psychochemical cure for schizophrenia has been abandoned by most medical researchers.

LSD proved to be a most useful tool in work with schizophrenic children. The response of autistic children (those with little or no awareness of their environment) who were treated with LSD greatly encouraged therapists in the field. They made contact with patients they were never able to reach before.

A recent case in point in a New York State mental institution showed that the reactions of the adult schizophrenic to psychedelic drugs were not typical for the autistic schizophrenic child.

Dr. Lauretta M. Bender of Creedmore State Hospital, Long Island, New York, administered the drug to vegetablelike autistic children who were unable to give or receive affection, enjoy the world around them, or even play. She also administered the drug to schizophrenic children who had withdrawn into a world of fantasy. In both cases she recorded improvement in behavioral patterns and in response to the environment. The children also seemed more relaxed and showed more alert facial expressions, smiled, and frowned, while some even attempted to relate to others. The common symptom in such youngsters of beating their heads against walls decreased dramatically; eating and sleeping habits improved, and for the first time they showed some ability to communicate with the nurses and doctors about them.

Another case on the records reports the LSD treatment of a pair of five-year-old twins who had almost completely withdrawn from human contact. After the drug was administered, the twins markedly reduced their bizarre repetitive movements and mechanical rhythmic activities; for the first time there were signs that they might be reached.

The report on the case stated, "One reason why childhood autism has been so resistant to treatment is that its victims can make no contact or express any interest in the people who try to help them. There is little eye contact, no speech, lack of concentration on everything but mechanically repeated activities." LSD broke down this pattern with the result that the twins displayed a marked improvement in their social behavior.

LSD has been a very useful psychotherapeutic tool in treatment of the classic neuroses. According to Dr. Sidney Cohen, Chief of the Division of Narcotics Addiction and Drug Abuse of the National Institute of Mental Health in Bethesda, Maryland, one such application of the drug showed improvements that he has summarized in the following statement:

> (1) They reduce the patient's defensiveness and allow repressed memories and conflictual material to come forth. The recall of these events is improved and the abreaction is intense.
> (2) The emerging material is better understood because the patient sees the conflict as a visual image, or in vivid visual symbols. It is accepted without being overwhelming because the detached state of awareness makes the emerging guilt feeling less devastating.
> (3) The patient feels closer to the therapist and it is easier for him to express irrational feelings.
> (4) Alertness is not impaired and insights are retained after the drug has worn off.

These dramatic results have convinced many psychotherapists that LSD helps therapy to proceed at a much faster rate than it ordinarily would. Some spectacular and almost unbelievable progress has actually been achieved with only one dose of the drug.

In an article entitled "The Curious Story Behind the New Cary Grant," *Look* Magazine described how psychotherapy with LSD had removed many stumbling blocks from the path of the star's personal happiness and fulfillment. The popular actor confided to his interviewer that he had in the past been emotionally immature, painfully shy, egocentric, and at fault for the failure of his three marriages. In just weeks of therapy, he found "all the loose ends of my life knitting together" and his "last defense" crumbling.

The success of the therapy, taken under the guidance of Dr. Mortimer Hartman, a West Coast psychiatrist who has submitted a medical paper on the Cary Grant and Betsy Drake case and his effective treatment of 112 other patients, made Grant a "zealous missionary" for the clinical use of LSD.

"All my life, I've been searching for peace of mind," he was quoted in *Look*. "I'd explored yoga and hypnotism and made attempts at mysticism. Nothing really seemed to give me what I wanted until this treatment . . .

". . . I've been going around in a fog. You're just a bunch of molecules until you know who you are . . . To my delight, I found I had a tough inner core of strength. In my youth, I was very dependent . . . Now people come to me for help!"

Betsy Drake, his wife at the time, told the *Look* reporter, that her LSD therapy not only relieved her of harrowing memories as a survivor of the *Andrea Doria* sinking, but helped her to make "the painful decision" to leave her husband, who then really "wanted to be free."

"You learn to die under LSD," she explained. "You face up to all the urges in you—love, sex, jealousy, the wish to kill . . ."

Questioned about his relationship with women, Grant was quoted, at the time as follows: "My relations with women will be different. I used to love a woman with great passion, and we destroyed each other. Or I loved not at all or in friendship. Now I'm ready to love on an equal level . . . All my life I think I've been running away from what I wanted most . . ."

Patients from all walks of life echo Grant's praise for the experimental form of psychotherapy. One such case on record relates how the senior executive of an international communications agency had undergone four years of analysis, four days a week. He said that a few LSD sessions had given him more insight into his personality than the whole of his four years in analysis. He indicated that he could ill afford to spend endless hours in psychoanalytic sessions and, in view of his failure to improve under orthodox analysis, he gave up this method in preference to LSD sessions.

Psychiatrists have admitted that what may require a year in verbal analysis of the patient's neuroses can be achieved in a few sessions with LSD. This is mainly attributed to the drug's effect that allows the psychic material to merge into consciousness where it would normally be shut out. More extreme cases are equally susceptible to LSD treatment as recent reports on homosexuals and alcoholics indicate.

LSD psychotherapy of alcoholism has been more successful than any other method used in the past. There are five million alcoholics in the United States and the recovery rate without treatment is four percent—a very low figure indeed. With LSD psychotherapy the number of recoveries have soared to as high as fifty percent.

The procedure in using LSD as a cure for alcoholics differs slightly from ordinary psychedelic therapy. Although a great many alcoholics were willing to try the drug as a cure, there have been conspicuous difficulties in getting the therapists to agree that this method had merit. The theory among those who tried to aid alcoholics was that the drunk must hit bottom before he can be saved. The opponents of LSD therapy claimed that the imitation delirium tremens created by the drug would be of no value since most of the patients' case histories were replete with entries of real d.t.'s that had been experienced repeatedly without any beneficial results whatsoever. The advocates of LSD in alcoholic therapy argued that the patient's hitting bottom was only significant if it created a realization on his part that he was destroying himself and could not continue in this manner any longer. The patient at this point, they added, had to admit without pulling any punches that he was a confirmed alcoholic.

These therapists conceded that there had been no change in the patients who had suffered the actual delirium tremens, but they attributed this to their refusal to admit certain truths about their alcoholic condition. LSD, they claimed, would not only produce an imitation delirium tremens, but would also break down whatever ego defenses the patient still had, thus creating in him a greater awareness of his situation with the subsequent realization that he was in serious need of help. They were certain that LSD would assist in destroying the alcoholic's previous behavioral patterns so that he might rebuild more sociably acceptable norms.

To test the hypothesis, they calculated that a more-than-average dose would be necessary to break down any resistance the patient might have to the drug. That is why the dose commonly used in alcoholic therapeutic programs today is much higher than the 100 to 250 micrograms used by the average tripper. It is usually between 300 to 800 micrograms and is administered only once or twice in the belief that the profound experience would be of sufficient force to detour the alcoholic from his destructive path.

Although not all the initial results from LSD therapy for alcoholics were successful, some outstanding ones were recorded and these were considered enough to justify further use. As mentioned before, most of the early work with LSD in this type of therapy was done in Canada. In one experiment at the Saskatchewan Hospital, Drs. Hoffer and Osmond deliberately chose twenty-four of the most intractable alcoholics they could find in their own as well as other hospitals and agencies throughout the country. In the inquiry they sent out, they made clear what they were seeking. "We want your worst cases. We are not interested in mild cases that could recover through Alcoholics Anonymous or through any other agencies that you now have available."

Among the subjects accepted for this experiment, the average period of uncontrolled drinking spanned twelve years; one-third of the subjects had experienced the d.t.'s and ninety percent of the group had tried Alcoholics Anonymous with no results. They all had serious personality disorders, half of the group having been diagnosed as psychopaths and four being actual psychotics. The success of a group with this particular make-up was spectacular. Six of the twenty-four subjects have been completely abstinent since cessation of the treatment. Another six showed definite reduction in alcoholic intake. The remaining twelve were unchanged. In a group of this sort, a fifty-percent success rate is indeed impressive.

This Canadian program, after thirteen years of dealing with more than eight hundred hard-core alcoholics published a report of the results:

> When psychedelic therapy is given to alcoholics, about one-third will remain sober after the therapy is completed and another one-third will be benefited. If schizophrenics and malverians

> [people with a biochemical aberration that makes them respond poorly or not at all to the psychedelic experience] are excluded from LSD therapy, the results should be better by about thirty percent. There are no published papers using psychedelic therapy which show it does not help about fifty percent of the treated group. Our conclusion after 13 years of research is that, properly used, LSD therapy can turn a large number of alcoholics into sober members of society. Even more important, this can be done very quickly and therefore very economically; whereas with standard therapy one bed might be used to treat about four to six patients per year, with LSD, one can easily treat up to 36 patients per bed, per year.

Allowing for all these variables, the success in keeping alcoholics sober for long periods is greater than that shown by any other drug treatment or such group-support activities as conducted by Alcholics Anonymous. In contrast to the almost fifty percent aided by LSD therapy, Dr. J. Ross Maclean, Medical Director of Hollywood Hospital in British Columbia, said that only five to ten percent abstinence has been achieved by other drug and psychotherapeutic methods.

Dr. Osmond attributed the success of the LSD therapy to the premise that "alcoholics are quite setbound. But an overwhelming experience, such as LSD provides, may break through the alcoholics's rigidified notion of himself. It's a matter of getting a sufficiently vivid experience so that they don't deny what has happened but incorporate it into themselves."

Dr. Sanford Unger, Chief of Psychological Research at the Spring Grove State Hospital, explains that LSD induces an emotional re-education of the patient, something that other therapists have found almost impossible to achieve with the more familiar types of psychotherapy.

Alcoholism, according to Dr. Unger, has produced changes in the personality of the subjects that have completely alienated them from society:

> What we are trying to do with the help of LSD, is reverse this 10- to 12-year pathological process and start a new set of feelings and attitudes which will point the patient in a direction where there is some possibility for growth and personal satisfaction. It has long been known that profound negative or so-called traumatic experiences have a long-term wake of negative consequences, such as neuroses based on childhood experience, but

until LSD it was very difficult to create the same cause-effect relationship with profoundly positive experiences.

A federally backed program for research into LSD therapy for alcoholics in the United States has been established on the basis of the encouraging results recorded by the therapists in Canada. Even the federal hospital at Lexington, Kentucky, which specifically treats addicts to the hard narcotics, at one time attempted to use LSD in therapy programs.

It is clear that the promise of LSD may be as infinite as the experience itself.

CHAPTER NINETEEN

A LOVE DRUG: LSD AND SEX

From Frigidity to the Marriage Bed

For many of the same reasons that LSD is employed as a therapeutic tool in the treatment of psychoses, neuroses, and alcoholism, it is being used to combat marital problems—frigidity in women, impotence in men, homosexuality, and other sexual aberrations. But despite Dr. Timothy Leary's claim of women experiencing thousands of orgasms in a single sexual encounter under the influence of LSD, the drug itself is neither an aphrodisiac nor an anaphrodisiac.

Scientists are virtually unanimous in agreeing that LSD is not a "sex drug," although it can act as an emotional relaxant and strong stimulus in a sexual encounter. If the couple under LSD has sexual engagement in mind, then LSD can influence the experience just as it can influence any other area of activity. If the setting is right, and the partners are compatible, the experience has been said to be indescribably ecstatic.

The theory behind its use as a therapeutic tool in sexual problems is much the same as that of other psychedelic therapy. Many of the traumas involved in sexual inversions are swept away and the subject is forced to come face to face with the truth presented under psychedelic influence. If, however, the subject cannot reach to the bottom of his or her disorder, then the problem cannot even begin to be cured. Like the "hitting-bottom" theory in alcoholism therapy, recognition of the problem is an important first step, and LSD seems to first define the problem and then dissolve it.

Aside from the heterosexual subjects who occasionally fear an expression of latent homosexuality in innocent displays of affection to others of the same sex during the psychedelic session, the majority of reports about LSD therapy in solving sexual problems have been encouraging.

The problems of alienation and loneliness that lead many to extremely introverted behavior with the resulting breakdown in family relationships, has put LSD to work as a marriage counselor. The current rate of divorce, separation, and marriages strained by incompatability betrays the dismal fact that there is something vitally lacking in the husband-wife relationship. Realizing this, Dr. Richard Alpert has included in his book, *LSD,* co-authored with Sidney Cohen, a chapter entitled, "A Manual for Making the Marriage New."

The LSD experience, he states, will throw new light on the partnership, restore appreciation for the partner, and open the doors to a new evaluation of the complete relationship. It will also allow, he says, for successful marital adjustments and help people overcome their problems of alienation.

The sexual relations of the partners in marriage are, of course, of prime importance to the union. In the following case history, the husband had "simply lost interest" in the relationship:

> Our marriage had been relatively stable for six years and we had been blessed with three children—two boys and a girl. However, there came a point when I found myself bored with the children and I thought my wife paid too much attention to them. I slowly began losing interest in having sexual relations with her and started spending the weekends out with the boys and staying in the city late instead of heading for home after the day's work at the office was done.
>
> After about six months of that sort of behavior, things began to disintegrate. I found myself staying away from home overnight. I would stay at a hotel in the city—and the idea entered my mind of seeking other sexual partners aside from my wife. At the same time, my wife and I began having frequent quarrels. She suffered sudden fits of crying and, since this whole experience of marital disintegration was alien to me, my work at the office began to be affected and I became dissatisfied with my job. I also experienced a considerable amount of guilt in the extra-

marital relationships I was carrying on at the time. After one of our disputes at home we agreed to go to a marriage counselor. When that proved ineffective, he recommended that we consult a psychiatrist.

The psychiatrist did not seem to view our problem as a very serious one, and after a few sessions, he suggested LSD. I had, of course, heard of LSD through reading a number of magazine articles, and was against the idea. He carefully explained the real facts about the drug and put our minds at ease. He suggested that I undergo the LSD treatment first. After the LSD experience the doctor gave me a tranquilizer and sent me home to my wife.

The experience was unbelievable and I remember it vividly to this day. I came home, sat in the living room and watched my wife going about her everyday duties concerning the children. The experience I had undergone in the psychiatrist's office made me realize that the attitudes I held toward my wife and the children were related to my own childhood.

I had been an only child and attention had been plentiful. I realized that when the children had been a bit younger I had been free with my affection toward them. Somewhere along the way, however, I began to feel that I was in competition with them for my wife's love. I realized it was an infantile reaction to deny my wife sexual relations as a way of punishment.

I sat there for an hour watching my wife's actions, and was overwhelmed by the affection and love she displayed toward the family. It paralleled and even exceeded the love displayed by my own mother and father. Suddenly I was overwhelmed by love for her that I had never felt before. It was an even stronger emotion than the love I felt for her before we were married. A calm mood descended over me and I felt thankful to the doctor for the opportunity he had given me to experience the LSD situation. . . .

The case history goes on to state that the problem was completely resolved. Not only did the patient require no further LSD sessions, but the follow-up revealed that he had gained many other useful insights into his work and his life as a whole through the experience. The feeling of love felt by the patient on returning home after the session was also translated into sensual terms when the subject and his wife went to bed that evening. The patient states that the experience was exhilarating.

"I found that having sexual intercourse with my wife was as new and beautiful and exciting as the first time. I couldn't imagine that only a few months ago I had been trying to avoid her, never realizing until I took LSD what the relationship really meant to me."

As has been explained, LSD is not an aphrodisiac but since the primary effects of the drug heighten the perceptions, it follows that the pleasure derived from sexual activity may also likely be increased. In the preceding case, however, there was no sexual problem. What the LSD session did was to make clear to the husband that his reactions to his wife constituted infantile and immature behavior. Once the true reasons for his actions were clarified, he was able not only to continue the relationship but to see it with new eyes. It gives ample evidence that a drug used in this psychosexual area can be useful in uncovering the true self, exposing the behavioral patterns for what they are, giving the subject a truer insight into his personality.

Those who use their jobs, economic position, status, or other social attainments to sublimate their sex drive are deprived of fraudulent defenses under the stimulus of LSD, which makes them realize that their preoccupations were at the expense of other equally, if not more, meaningful experiences. Their behavioral patterns are clearly visible as such and a more realistic appraisal of the self usually follows.

More serious sexual conditions have also been aided by LSD. Frigidity, a problem that showed invariably poor results in attempted cures, was the subject of a book by Constance Newland: *Myself and I*. At the time the book was published in 1962, such uses for LSD were relatively unexplored. Miss Newland (a pseudonym), who had been undergoing psychotherapy for some years without any progress at all, agreed to try LSD. She had already reached the point where she was prepared to accept her problem and live with it for, as she states, she knew "that frigidity among women is almost as prevalent as the common cold and just about as incurable." Her particular position in society enabled her to continue and function as usual and to sublimate her condition through her work. The results of her twenty-five LSD sessions were so successful that she published a book in which she described the experience in detail.

In *Myself and I* she explains that after the death of her husband she tried to bury herself in her career. Aware of her problem, she sought help in psychoanalysis but it failed to elicit a conscious image of her condition. The method also failed to successfully conjure up childhood memories and experiences—a necessary step that enables the patient to come to new terms with problems deeply rooted in the past. LSD does just those things; it not only presents the patient's problems but yields probably the most vivid account possible of those past events that must be dealt with to begin to effect any type of cure.

During her sessions, Miss Newland experienced a number of clear images of her frigidity. She felt herself symbolically turned to ice; her teeth chattered and her body trembled. She visualized a white marble statue of a nude woman with two gaping holes in the place where the breasts should have been. She also re-experienced several traumatic incidents of childhood that had long been repressed in her subconscious. By reliving them she was able to slough off all the sexual inhibitions that had prevented her from living a normal life.

"As a baby," she writes, "I had seen the act of intercourse which then appeared to be an act of violence in which father 'choked' mother. That scene had so alarmed and sickened me that, as a protection, I had determined never to feel anything so that I would not be hurt."

She then goes on to explain in detail the one childhood experience that was most responsible for her problem.

"At long, long last, I had uncovered the classic Freudian trauma responsible for my sexual difficulty: one too strong, too hot enema, received when I was two-and-a-half years old. It was preposterous, but undeniable. At the age of two-and-a-half, my ego was helpless and could only fend off the problem by repression, which later turned out to be ineffective and involved the permanent hindrance to further development—of frigidity."

LSD enabled Miss Newland to focus on those mental and emotional experiences that had long been unavailable to her conscious inspection. As a matter of fact, she admits becoming aware of her "subconscious" for the first time since what it contained was so repellent to her that she had refused to allow any of it to emerge into her conscious mind. By being able to examine these unpleasant elements and see them for what they were, she succeeded in dismissing them.

Other cases involving frigidity were reported by Drs. Thomas Ling and John Buckman working at the Marlboro Day Hospital in London, England. In the *Psychedelic Review,* they published a report of sixteen cases they treated successfully with LSD therapy. LSD, they write, is able to effect the cure through the recovery of early sexual fantasies or traumatic experiences responsible for the symptom formation.

One of the patients reported a complete lack of sexual desire although she was married and had two children. Through the LSD sessions, she was able to recover memories of her father who showed absolutely no interest in her and of an early attempted rape by her young uncle while she was just a child. These unpleasant recollections had completely escaped her memory and their subsequent retrieval enabled her to change her view toward sex. A month later, she was able to report. "After the last treatment, I had my first intercourse with full orgasm internally which was a completely new and wonderful experience. My sexual life is now completely different and I get a wonderful feeling out of it on most occasions. The marriage is now very much better, but I believe there is still room for improvement."

Another case involves a twenty-six-year-old girl from India who was living in London and wanted to marry but was afraid she would be unable to have sexual relations. After her LSD sessions, she, too, unearthed childhood memories through which she was able to understand her sexual fears. The tensions she had with respect to establishing sexual contact vanished and she felt a new emotional freedom. She told the doctors that after her treatment, she was "able to get full satisfaction out of sexual intercourse and always achieved full orgasm."

Homosexuality has similarly shown to be tractable through LSD therapy. By defining the anxiety, unconscious blocks, fears, and inhibitions, the drug has succeeded in resolving the feelings of guilt involved in the aberration and allowed deviates to accept the problem with a greater degree of confidence. In other individuals, it has opened up these areas for renewed inspection, involving the subject in heterosexual behavior.

In like manner LSD has been useful in the treatment of other inversions—fetishism, transvestism, and sadomasochism. Because these sexual disorders are locked in the same subconcious to which LSD seems to hold a key, doctors see great hope in the use of psychedelics for further treatment of such aberrations along similar lines. According to Masters and Houston, ". . . these drugs are so interesting and promising they should be thoroughly explored in this connection."

SECTION THREE:

THE AMPHETAMINES

CHAPTER TWENTY

SPEED KILLS: THE ABUSE OF AMPHETAMINES

New Labs--the Family Medicine Cabinet, the Garden, and the Supermarket

Dozens of other drugs have come to the fore along with marijuana and LSD. They, too, have risen up from the fringe elements of American society to become middle-class household words. Most of them, of course, do not carry the taboos associated with marijuana and LSD. Stimulants, depressants, tranquilizers, sleeping pills, and any other variety of chemical compound that can cause or change a mood, have been absorbed into the nation's pharmacopoeia. Copping pills, swallowing capsules, downing tablets have become a national habit. Apart from the seventy million American consumers of alcohol—five million of whom, by conservative estimate, are alcoholics—another fifteen million take amphetamine (speed); thirty million use barbiturates (sleeping pills); twelve million use tranquilizers; while an untold number of youngsters sniff glue, drink codeine-based cough medicine, and will try any new mind-altering substance that comes along. In addition, there are an estimated fifty thousand heroin addicts who appear to be beyond redemption.

Today's youngsters can hardly be blamed for the wave of drug use now sweeping the country. Most of them first witnessed the emergence of mind-altering substances in the fifties as their parents took eagerly to the huge variety of new drugs affecting the psyche that became popular after World War II.

The amphetamines—particularly benzedrine, which was perfected during the war—began to be used as a stimulant and everyday "pick-me-up." And then along came Miltown—the first of the host of tranquilizers that were to follow. By that time barbiturates were already being swallowed in increasing quantities. It was not uncommon for parents to dose their children with half a barbiturate tablet so that they would be sure to go to sleep.

Some children were thus reared on a diet of mood-altering drugs along with Wheaties and sundaes. If they did not actually swallow these compounds as children, they still had ample opportunity to witness their parents' indulgence in them. The result is visible today—an unparalleled rise in drug use and abuse that has become an increasing worry of medical authorities and social legislators alike.

As teen-agers, these children of the drug age soon took their own independent look into their parents' medicine chest, discovering a cornucopia of vials and bottles offering instant relief from reality. Pills, powders, leaves, fungi, liquids, and seeds—both natural and synthetic—were being added to constantly by naturalists and pharmacologists, while the publicity showered upon the subject in the popular media hardly toned down the curiosity they had aroused.

The tranquilizer-amphetamine-barbiturate boom that began in the early fifties (over twelve thousand patents for these drugs were filed up to 1967) demonstrates the immense following these drugs have attracted to their fold. The expansion of pharmacology and biochemistry was so great after the war that the textbooks dealing with these subjects were being constantly revised as dozens of new drugs were thrown on the market monthly.

Substances widely used today were still unknown only a few years ago and, until recently, many drugs now widely accepted were not yet recognized or understood. A good many of the new drugs were a boon to the psychologists and psychiatrists in the treatment of mental disorders. The average man and woman, unable to cope adequately with the pressures of modern living, received them with equal enthusiasm.

Although the older generation adhered mainly to the sleeping pill-tranquilizer syndrome, their children were more curious about the other substances they had heard about. Students on high school and college campuses across the nation made good use of the facilities at hand to discover the latest ripple in mind-altering substances. They learned that if they could not always obtain a drug directly, there was always some underground method of accomplishing this end. They read avidly about the "magic" mushrooms, peyote, mescaline, and psilocybin—hallucinogens milder than LSD. They began writing letters to garden-supply houses and purchasing "peyote buttons," which they would chew for psychedelic effects. They discovered that nutmeg contains a small percentage of hallucinogenic matter that produces the psychedelic flash.

Their curiosity about mind-altering substances was almost as zealous as that of the scientists filing their research reports on the subject. They discovered the effects of sniffing airplane glue, and the flashback-type of high from sniffing the fumes of paint thinner and cleaning fluid. All three—airplane glue, paint thinner, and cleaning fluid—contain a chemical to induce rapid evaporation in the compound. Youngsters quickly caught on to its properties and eagerly bought up any commercial mixture containing the intoxicating substance. There was a question at one time of eliminating this chemical from the market but it is so widely used in industry that the attempt was soon abandoned. Most youngsters quickly learned, however, that this practice is extremely dangerous and can cause serious damage to such organs as the kidneys and liver. Since there is no way to regulate the dosage, such indulgence not infrequently ends in dizziness or unconsciousness, sometimes resulting in a fatal coma.

Another popular "kick" is the use of codeine-based cough medicine. Codeine, one of the milder derivatives of opium, is an exempt narcotic—a prescription is not needed for its acquisition. In some states where its use is restricted, a substitute synthetic codeine is usually available in most drugstores, where young people buy it for lack of the availability of more potent drugs.

Youngsters are not the only ones familiar with the properties of cough medicine; heroin addicts also use it as a substitute when they cannot get the stronger drug. Although addiction is rare, there is an element of danger involved in sustained use. It is still being used to turn on, however, and some hippies develop a phony cough and dash down to their neighborhood pharmacist for a supply.

Belladonna and amylnitrite have also been picked up by the drug generation in recent years. Belladonna is available in various patent medicines for asthma and is quite legal. One such mixture which comes in a thick green syrup is unbearably bitter and excessive use commonly results in nightmare experiences. Nagging nausea, exhaustion, restlessness, and loss of motor facilities are other adverse effects that commonly follow an overdose.

Amylnitrite vials, called "snappers," are especially popular with youngsters when they are already high on one of the hallucinogens. This drug is a legal prescription for heart condition and asthma, speeding up the circulation and thus increasing the effects of the psychedelic drug previously ingested. The effects last only for a few minutes or so, providing an extra fillip to the psychedelic drug.

Hippies avail themselves of the research reports of naturalists and pharmacologists filed in local libraries. They are quick to appropriate such findings. For example, the flowers of the Scotch Broom plant—a plant that grows extensively along highways and in empty fields—were also discovered to be a good substitute for marijuana. Another recent discovery reported that Hawaiian woodflowers were psychedelic. Similarly, periwinkle leaves were found to produce a high if the dried and shredded leaves are smoked like marijuana. The plant with its blue blossoms is common throughout the United States, and the reports of its effects claim that "the world was viewed as through the wrong end of a telescope."

Medical reports describe periwinkle as containing the source of vincristine and vinblastine—two potent drugs used in the treatment of acute leukemia and Hodgkin's disease. There is no certainty, however, whether these two drugs are the cause of the psychedelic effects of smoking the periwinkle leaves. A chemist at Eli Lilly and Company, an Indianapolis firm that manufactures the drugs, reported that they are highly unstable and probably do not get into the smoke of burning periwinkle leaves in an active form. Nevertheless, the chemist was quick to point out that "periwinkle, like most inedible plants, is toxic. You might get pretty sick to your stomach."

The ingenuity of youngsters in constantly finding new trip tickets borders on the miraculous. Quick-freeze aerosol spray is one of the latest means they have discovered for freaking out. In October, 1967, one of the national magazines carried the tragic story of a seventeen-year-old New York suburbanite who inhaled the fumes from an aerosol can of cocktail-glass chiller as a way to turn on. When he gave it to his eleven-year-old sister, she immediately lost consciousness and three minutes later died from asphyxiation. Such are the perils of Freon-12, an odorless, colorless cryogenic gas that obtains its lethal effect from freezing the larynx and thus cutting off oxygen to the lungs. Yet, hippies and college students were still turning to it despite doctors' warnings that sniffers were liable to risk brain damage from anoxia. Even while the second victim—an Oregon high-school student—fell to the deadly gas, a medical investigator reported the rapid disappearance of the quick-freeze spray from the shelves of Portland supermarkets.

The most powerful of all the new drugs is STP, said to be far stronger than LSD. Supposedly named after the oil additive used by auto racers, it acts instantly with a veritable vortex of vivid and often horrifying hallucinations that may last for as long as three or four days. Hippies are the most frequent users of this drug. When it first became popular, at least a dozen of San Francisco's Haight-Ashbury residents found themselves being rushed to hospitals as the result of bum trips.

The danger of such unfortunate endings to the STP experience lies in the particular constituents of the drug that make it impervious to the usual antidotes employed against the bad effects of LSD. Tranquilizers, sedatives, and other central-nervous-system depressants that exert a calming influence on the LSD high only tend to aggravate the bad side effects of STP.

STP was recently identified by the federal government as 2,5-Dimethoxy-4-methyl-amphetamine. It tends to impair breathing and produce an irregular heartbeat. Thus when chlorpromazine or sedatives are taken by STP users they tend to increase the undesirable effects and the subsequent damage to the nerves may cause death.

Sandoz Pharmaceuticals (the developers of LSD) opened an interesting social perspective with the discovery of "quickie" trips supplied by a series of tryptamines—drugs with effects similar to LSD but that can be spaced for almost any length of time according to the user's desire. DMT (Dimethyltryptamine), the quickest of the new line, has been available for some time on the black market. It is popular among drug users across the nation who smoke it like marijuana by mixing it with parsley leaves. The effects come quickly—hallucinations follow within a few seconds.

Although the DMT experience is short-lived, with an effective range from fifteen minutes to half an hour, the sensation is so powerful that DMT has in a short time become a favorite staple of the drug culture. Its unusual properties have earned it the nicknames, the "lunch-hour special" and "the commuter's jet."

Another factor that has served to endear this drug to a considerable number of people is its comparatively simple manufacturing process. Although LSD can be made inexpensively, its production still calls for a small but intricate panoply of equipment and know-how. DMT, on the other hand, requires no more elaborate paraphernalia than a spoon, a stove, and filter papers. Obtaining its ingredients poses no particular problem since each has a half-dozen industrial uses that make them readily available on the open market. As a result, underground manufacturers have wasted no time in adding the drug to their list of products.

This trend of sub rosa drug production has not escaped the government watchdogs. Testifying before a Senate subcommittee on the flood of novel substances emerging from the laboratory, Dr. Stanley Yolles, Director of the National Institute of Mental Health, predicted that in the next five to ten years we will have a hundredfold increase in drugs that affect the mind.

CHAPTER TWENTY-ONE

METHEDRINE: THE SUPERMAN DRUG

"If Mother Uses It, Can It Be So Bad?"

Perhaps the most widespread of the new drugs in the underground culture is the stimulant known as "speed." The term usually refers to the stimulant, methamphetamine hydrochloride, best-known by one of its trade names, methedrine (also termed "crystal" by users because it comes in crystalline form). Speed may also refer to the complete amphetamine family of drugs to which methedrine belongs. The nickname is derived from the drug's fast-acting effects and striking reactions on the human nervous system.

Other names for the amphetamines themselves are many and varied. Because their effects keep the user alert and active and ward off sleep, they were once known as "pep pills," but a whole lexicon of new derivatives has been coined for them as well—bennies, bombitas, copilots, footballs, lid proppers, wake-ups, eyeopeners, truckdrivers, cartwheels, coast-to-coasts, purple hearts, dexies, and splash. The slang names usually come from the various effects, the purposes to which the drug is put, or from the trade names of the manufacturers.

Thus "bennie" is derived from benzedrine; "dexie" from dexedrine; "meth" from methedrine; "black bombers" from the form of amphetamine that is manufactured in the shape of small black pills; the term "purple hearts" is similarly derived from the shape and color of the pills. "Copilots," "truckdrivers," "cartwheels," and "coast-to-coasts" originate with the habit of truck-drivers using speed to stay awake on long overnight hauls.

Amphetamine, first prepared in 1887, was not synthesized until 1927 in the form of amphetamine sulphate (benzedrine), at which time it became a substitute for the drug ephedrine. During the Spanish Civil War it was placed in ships' survival packs. Almost simultaneously it was issued to German paratroopers for routine operational use. Its first important medical application came with the treatment of narcolepsy (the inability to stay awake) in the thirties. In 1931 it was issued for public sale in drugstores in the United States as an ingredient in inhalers for relief of common colds and stuffy noses. It soon became apparent that the drug could also be used as a stimulant. As a result, the Food and Drug Administration put immediate pressure on the manufacturers to withdraw the use of this substance in cold remedies.

Stimulants received their greatest boost during World War II when troops, availing themselves of the newly developed synthetics, stayed on the battlefield in a condition that, without such drugs, would have sent them staggering from exhaustion to their sleeping bags. American and German pilots soon began packing vials of the tiny pills along with the other necessities for survival. The German pilots were inveterate pill chewers as they flew their bombers over England.

In the rush to develop new weapons during the war, German and American scientists kept awake over their highly secret research by using amphetamines in copious quantities. Both sides swallowed millions of tablets during this period, and their use was crucial in the feats of soldiers who would otherwise have been too fatigued to pull through many a hard-fought campaign.

After the war two new amphetamines were developed—dextro-amphetamine sulphate (dexedrine) and methamphetamine hydrochloride (methedrine). Today there are dozens of brands of amphetamines legally available in the United States.

Amphetamines have been called the "superman drug" for the simple reason that one of their effects gives the user an illusory sense of power and well-being. Early pharmacological studies reaffirmed the fact that they considerably raised the capacity to perform physical and mental tasks. An increase in intelligence by an average of up to eight points was reported by Drs. William Sargant and J. M. Blackburn in the British medical journal, *Lancet*. Other more complex activities, however, like driving a car or playing a game of cards, remain qualitatively unaffected although their duration may be sustained longer than would normally be the case.

A host of problems was encountered in the early research on the pharmacology of the drug. In his book *Crime and Personality,* published by Routledge and Kegan Paul, London, 1964, H. J. Eysenck described the hypnotics (drugs such as barbiturates) as having effects similar to alcohol and directly contrary to those of the stimulants—caffeine, amphetamine, and cocaine. In the personality pendulum swinging from introversion to extroversion, he found that hypnotics direct a given personality toward extroversion while stimulants thrust the individual toward introversion.

In other words, a stimulant by prodding the mind causes introversion (fewer external stimuli are needed to set the brain patterns in motion); hypnotics, on the other hand, dull the activity of the mind and cause extroversion (more external stimuli are required to set the psyche working). Thus, pot—a stimulant—makes even small things seem significant and thereby reduces the need for external action; alcohol, a hypnotic, is action-oriented because it feeds on external stimuli.

The aforegoing may seem contrary to many of the opinions generally held about drug effects. The hyperactive and talkative person high on amphetamines gives the appearance of being extroverted rather than introverted. His thought patterns, however, are directed inward toward the self, rather than outward to the environment. Barbiturates, on the other hand, channel the reactions outward to the immediate surroundings.

Surprising as it may seem, the extrovert is ruled by inhibitory factors; he constantly needs new stimuli and is subsequently easily bored, with the result that he appears more extroverted than the introvert who has low inhibition and therefore has an increased capacity for accommodating the same stimulus.

Inhibition serves as the gate that shelters the self from the outside world; any stimulus or activity produces inhibition and thus automatically pulls the gate shut. Protection from stimuli, Freud observed, was almost more important to an organism than their reception; and in *The Doors of Perception,* Aldous Huxley sees the mind as a huge valve to shut off experience. Amphetamines act as such a valve.

The discovery that amphetamines direct the personality pendulum toward introversion is underscored by the kinds of people who are the most ardent devotees of the drug. Tired housewives and teen-agers constitute groups who, besides needing energy for their often-exhausting activities, are also bored and starved for stimulation. Their reason for taking the drug usually centers around their urge to exploit the available stimuli to the fullest possible extent. A lowering of inhibitory factors making users of the drug more adaptable to the standards and behavior of those around them is another interesting effect, probably with a physiological basis.

The physical effects of the drug are exemplified by the speed freak (the heavy amphetamine user); they include dryness of the mouth and throat and wide-open eyes. Indeed, constant licking of dry lips and eyelids propped as wide as possible as though not being able to see well enough are the telltale signs by which a person shows the effects of amphetamines. Although the user commonly experiences a lift in spirits and a feeling of confidence, the side effects of the drug when taken in large doses range from insomnia and aggressiveness to touches of paranoia, especially with the eventual come-down. As the drug's effects subside most users complain of the shakes and nausea.

Despite a varied fluctuation of effects depending on the type of amphetamine, the dosage, and the length of time they are taken—as well as the individual user's physical and psychological state at any given time—the drug generally stimulates the mind, buoys the spirits, and elevates the environmental mood by acting directly on the central nervous system. Other accompanying effects are a reduction in appetite, which has resulted in incorporation of this drug into several varieties of reducing pills. The overstimulated nervous system precludes sleep or else makes it extremely difficult.

The antidepressant and euphoriant action on melancholy and dispiritedness have earned a niche for the amphetamines as a therapeutic crutch in aiding depressed individuals. Research in this field was carried out during and after World War II when the drug's properties were extensively explored. Its usefulness in combating fatigue has already been noted, but its therapeutic applications are equally impressive, although the personality improvements are cut short by withdrawal of the drug.

One such example is illustrated by a patient whose outlook on life was one of despondence and unrelieved depression. He had lost his job through a complete loss of ambition. In addition, his wife had cracked under the strain of his withdrawal. He lived a feckless state of existence during which he spent most of his time staring out the living-room window. An hour after taking the drug prescribed by his physician, he became increasingly more attentive and talkative. After sustained treatment for three days, his spirits had buoyed significantly. He kept busy around the house and by the sixth day he was humming snatches of tunes and expressed a desire to look for a job. By the tenth day, his wife indicated that he had reached his usual, good-humored state, but a few days later, his spirits began to sag and the despondency once again set in.

Disturbed and delinquent youngsters have also benefited from the drug's aforementioned propensity to make users more adaptable to the norms of their environment. H. J. Eysenck, in *Crime and Personality,* describes experiments with a group of disturbed and alienated children in which they were treated with amphetamine in an institution. Significant improvements were observed during the period of benzedrine medication, with particularly important gains in sociability, cooperation, attention, and alertness. This type of therapy has recently been criticized on the grounds that amphetamines cannot be a "socializing" drug because in its use by delinquents at large no "personality improvements are observed." The drug's advocates contend that in conjunction with an effective combination of social and psychiatric guidance, it can be helpful.

Catatonic schizophrenia, with its general symptoms of passivity and dullness, showed surprising susceptibility to therapeutic amphetamine treatment. In one case the patient in question had deteriorated to what was described as a "vegetable" condition, refusing to do anything herself to the point where she had to be spoon fed. Delusions and auditory hallucinations were common experiences, although these disappeared with the application of benzedrine as medication. Shortly thereafter she was up and about, assisting in ward work and taking a serious interest in others. As a result of the side effects, however, she slept only a few hours each night and continued to be irritable and agitated. After three weeks, marked improvement set in; she took delight in her surroundings, spreading cheer and talking freely about herself. She readily agreed that her personality had changed for the better. But continued medication was necessary to maintain this state.

Another application was found in the treatment of delirium tremens. One patient, a chronic alcoholic who reported hallucinations of spiders and snakes crawling all over the room, often became so terrified of his visions that he frequently lost consciousness. Benzedrine usually helped revive him to the point where he felt secure and cheerful. After several such treatments he was considered cured and returned home.

Because of such cases there is no question among medical authorities that these drugs possess some value in the treatment of depressed states. The aforementioned condition called narcolepsy, in which the patient keeps falling asleep at inappropriate moments, lends itself particularly to such application. The irritating side effects of the drug have, however, somewhat proscribed its use as an antidepressant. The havoc it wreaks on the appetite and natural sleep, coupled with the feelings of anxiety resulting from the come-down have caused it to lose much of its euphoric reputation.

The stimulating effects of amphetamine are undoubtedly useful in a variety of ailments from minor depressions to barbiturate poisoning to narcolepsy. Nevertheless, because of the drug's popularity with general practitioners, the American Medical Association Drug Committee warned that "amphetamines are not a magic source of extra mental or physical energy; they serve only to push the user to a greater expenditure of his own resources, sometimes to a hazardous point of fatigue that is often not recognized."

Another problem involves the amphetamines' appetite-suppressing properties, which are behind the millions of prescriptions written each year for patients trying to lose weight. In many cases, though, the overweight patient is so taken by the stimulating effects of the pills that this becomes the overriding reason for using them. Many pharmacologists are convinced that the average physician prescribes the amphetamines too freely—perhaps because of an incomplete understanding of the deleterious effects—and that people resort to them much too liberally.

Drs. I. Oswald and V. R. Thackore writing in the *British Medical Journal,* deplore the readiness with which people turn to the amphetamines, believing that "therapeutic indications for amphetamine are today becoming vanishingly small: Diet is best for obesity, they are no use in endogenous depressions, and there are better things for narcolepsy. But like barbiturates they are used by general practitioners and psychiatric out-patient departments almost as placebos, simply to do something for the vague miseries that abound in our society."

But the misuse and abuse of the drug continues. In various tablet and capsule forms as well as alone and in combination with other drugs, the amphetamines are prescribed by the billions every year. And according to the Food and Drug Administration, billions more find their way onto the black market. They have always been popular with harried executives, shift workers, long-distance truckdrivers, students cramming for exams, athletes who want to improve their performance, people with weight problems, and the aforementioned bored housewives and teen-agers who use them for "kicks."

The history of misuse following the discovery by teen-agers that sniffing the inhalers was a stimulating experience winds its way from the custom of basketball players chewing a few tablets for extra energy, to race horses being "doped" for similar reasons, and students working on term papers.

Former Food and Drug Administration Commissioner George P. Larick pointed out that "misuse of barbiturates and amphetamines on a 'do-it-yourself' basis has contributed to the rising toll of death on our highways, juvenile delinquency, violent and bizarre crimes, suicides, and other forms of antisocial behavior."

One of the classic cases of amphetamine misuse was that of the long-haul truckdriver who climbed into the sleeping berth in the cab of his truck and dozed off without bothering to stop the vehicle. He smashed into several poles and the truck was all but demolished. The driver, who had been taking amphetamines for two days to keep awake, miraculously survived. He later informed the police that he was sure somebody else was driving the truck when he went to sleep. Thus, one of the nicknames for the drug—"copilot."

Teen-agers, with justifiable reason, have been singled out as the chief culprits in the abuse of the drug. The example set by parents, according to Dr. Arnold T. Mandell of UCLA, is often the catalyst that puts youngsters within reach of amphetamines.

"One of the characteristic rationalizations," he says, "is if mother is on it, can it be so bad?"

The fifties saw the spread of the drug among teen-agers since at that time it could still be purchased in many states without prescription at corner drugstores. Many teen-agers cultivated a wide correspondence with pen pals for the specific purpose of obtaining the drug through the mails from another state where it was legal.

These underground customers spawned the emergence of a black market that still does a brisk trade in supplying the demand. Youngsters began using the drug to extend and intensify the weekend as a period of escape from school, or just for kicks. Whereas beer and liquor had once been the staples of the weekend party, the greedy swallowing of amphetamine tablets became the "in" thing among the young. Frantic party crashing, hot rodding, and surfing safaris were intensified by the charged-up effects of the amphetamines. Just at that time go-go dancing in dim discotheques became the rage and many of the young dancing girls kept up their frenetic pace with the aid of these pills.

At the time a sympathetic ear to amphetamine use was shown in the *London Evening Standard*. Investigating the use of the drug by London teen-agers, the writer did not think the pills posed a particular threat to either the youngsters or society. The verdict came down unmistakably on the side of teen-agers and their problems:

> They are looking for, and getting, stimulation, not intoxication. They want greater awareness, not escape. And the confidence and articulacy that the drug of the amphetamine group gives them are quite different from the drunken rowdiness of previous generations on a night out. The important difference between "purple hearts" and alcohol is that for the first time people in the mass are experiencing a cerebral sensation. Not a physical one. "Purple hearts" taken in the quantity that most teen-agers take them—half a dozen to a dozen, to keep them going over the weekend and save them the expense of hotel rooms and food—are not specifically harmful.

More recent reports from England show that the author of the above report was somewhat overly optimistic. From the vast number of prescriptions written for amphetamines in England and America, it has been noted that amphetamine addiction is rooted to personality disorders rather than from exposure to the drugs at home or as the result of keeping bad company.

It is no wonder that many of the runaway youngsters parading the streets of hippie enclaves in our large cities are the heaviest users of amphetamines. Many of them are confused, unstable personalities who depend on the artificial charge of amphetamine to lead them into the kind of hectic round of social relationships they seem to need. The glitter of the cities never shines so bright as when filtered through the energy of a handful of pills. Many of the small-town youngsters lean on this crutch to pace them through the city's carrousel of delights for which they left their homes. One of those speed freaks, a newcomer from Minnesota to San Francisco's Haight-Ashbury scene, described his first experience with the pill:

> We were all hanging out in front of a supermarket on Haight Street when someone suggested we all go to a folk-rock club nearby. On the way I swallowed a few pills I'd been given earlier in the day. I didn't sleep for two days. Every time I felt the effect wear off I'd take a couple more. I just couldn't bear to come down. I felt on top of the world, talking a blue streak, singing, dancing, and laughing without ever feeling in the least tired. I'd never felt so good in my whole life . . .
>
> The come-down came two days later. I felt as if all the energy had drained out of my body and my head was filled with lead. I kept drinking cokes though I hadn't eaten all that time. My mouth was dry as leather and I couldn't think straight no matter how hard I tried. I just wanted to go to sleep and wake up feeling like my old self.

The biggest headache to medical authorities, as pointed out by Dr. David Smith's Medical Clinic for hippies in San Francisco, is the teen-agers' lack of discretion in their use of the drugs. They pay little attention to dosage and some munch enough of the pills to stagger through the days as mindless zombies, "falling out" (sleeping) here and there for short periods, eating little until their bodies have wasted to shadows of their former selves.

Teen-agers are not the only group guilty of amphetamine misuse. It may seem surprising to learn that housewives constitute a category of pill abusers that has become the bane of many a physician deluged with requests for "pick-me-ups" from the tired homemakers.

Many women who have regular jobs in addition to their housekeeping tasks are bolstered to a dangerous degree by a daily diet of amphetamines. A great number of cases have come to light in which the women have forged prescriptions after having exhausted the credulity of their physician. In a few instances such drug abuse has placed a tremendous strain on the family life, leading to a complete collapse of the home when the case turned serious enough for the mother to be sent to a hospital for a cure.

Women guilty of such abuse usually assert that the pills, aside from giving them the energy to perform their home tasks, make them much better-tempered with the children. However, the tragedy sets in when the women need more and more of the pills in order to produce the feelings of equanimity and cheerfulness they desire. It is then that the endless rounds to different doctors and the forged prescriptions begin.

As opposed to the barbiturates, the amphetamines do not induce true physical addiction, although a slight tolerance (the need for larger doses) is known to be a frequent result of regular use. There is no question that a person may develop a psychological dependence on them.

Quitting the amphetamine habit can be relatively easy, if accompanied only by a minimum of side effects—the worst of which is passing fits of anxiety. The most deceptive quality about the drug, however, is the lift in spirits and feeling of confidence it inspires. It is exactly this property that makes for the psychological dependence that often develops from frequent indulgence.

Although not physically addictive, amphetamine use—if indulgence is sustained over a period of time—produces a slight disturbance in the brain's electrical activity. The disturbance, however, is not accompanied by any marked change in mood or personality. If withdrawal symptoms do occur, they are part of the general effects of the come-down and vanish with the passage of time.

As has been mentioned previously, the basic reason for addiction lies in the personality of the addict. D. S. Bell and W. H.

Trethowan report in the *Journal of Nervous and Mental Diseases* on a study made seven years ago of fourteen patients with a history of dependence on the drug. They showed that eleven were notorious in their excessive use of other drugs, such as morphine, bromide, barbiturates, alcohol, and even caffeine. Clearly, these patients had a personality flaw that drew them to a dependence on any kind of drug.

Dependence in extreme cases can be properly described as addiction. Habituated users pop pills by the handful several times a day in quantities that could be lethal to less inured people. In situations of this kind the danger arises when, in order to derive a greater "kick," the speed freak starts hypo-ing the amphetamine directly into the veins. Such dependence can then be said to have shaded over into addiction.

An unfortunate element often intrudes in the practice of amphetamine users resorting to barbiturates to relieve the after-effects of the pep pills; similarly, barbiturate users sometimes take amphetamines to pull themselves through another day. Persons under constant stress are often the victims of this vicious barbiturate-amphetamine-barbiturate cycle. Matters frequently are further complicated when one preparation consisting of an amphetamine-barbiturate mixture produces a dependence that can easily progress to a genuine physical addiction to the barbiturate components.

Apart from exhaustion and the legal penalties incumbent on possession of the drug, habituation and psychosis are the chief dangers that accompany the indiscriminate use of amphetamines. They are often, but not always, found in association. A large-enough dose—fifty micrograms—or approximately ten benzedrine tablets—is considered sufficient to precipitate a psychosis lasting up to a week in any normal person, according to Dr. Philip H. Connell, noted British physician, writing in his book *Amphetamine Psychosis,* published by Chapman and Hill, London, 1958. Dr. Connell says that the "symptoms of the madness induced by prolonged overdoses of amphetamines are primarily of a paranoid psychosis with ideas of reference, delusions of persecution, auditory and visual hallucinations in a setting of clear consciousness, possibly indistinguishable from acute or chronic schizophrenia. The condition is treated by withdrawal of the drug and giving barbiturates; there is a high relapse rate and in the physical and mental depression after large doses suicide is common."

Connell, in a review of forty-six cases of psychoses, noted that sixty-six percent had been previously treated for psychiatric illness; twenty-six came from a background involving a history of alcoholism and psychiatric disturbances; and of the group using amphetamines, every one of the members had previously used some other drug or excessive alcohol.

One of Dr. Connell's cases involved a woman who spent a week walking about the city in a daze—supposedly searching for God. She began this "mission" because she had received special signs—after she had been taking dexedrine for weight reduction and fatigue. During the period of her wanderings she said that there were numerous symbolic meanings in incidents along the way that kept her going; she knew then that she was on the right track. But there were also persecutory figures in her experience that she believed were placed there to "test her." At the end of the period of her "search for God," she returned in a filthy state to the home of a relative where she proceeded to defecate on the rug.

Two other cases of the doctor's involved men who ingested the contents of amphetamine inhalers when they felt depressed. Both experienced feelings of paranoia. One hearing "pro" and "anti" voices felt that everyone was against him, even his wife. When she threatened to leave the house because of his strange behavior, he became acutely depressed and went to the hospital. The second man thought passersby looked at him in a strange way, and he began stalking the streets and sleeping in the park, where he discovered "gold" in the pebbles along the pathway. Eventually, he believed that the passersby were plotting to kill him and he tried to escape. Under the misapprehension that he was being followed by cars, he climbed to the roof of a building whence he began throwing roof tiles at his "persecutors."

Other research studies reveal that the hallucinations of schizophrenics are also markedly increased by use of amphetamines. A much smaller dose than is necessary to produce psychosis in normal people is adequate to produce psychotic reactions in schizophrenics, according to Connell. Therefore, a person with a body chemistry close to that of schizophrenics (frequently shown in previous abnormal behavior) needs only a relatively small dose of amphetamine to push him temporarily over the brink and into a psychotic state.

Before amphetamine inhalers were put on the restricted list, one could get a "charge" out of them that was one hundred times the clinical dose. Naturally, with such potency only a few sniffs away, it was no wonder that many a person with a precarious chemical balance went over the edge and found himself temporarily marooned in a psychotic state.

Adolescents, already troubled by crucial growing pains, also often experience psychotic reactions through amphetamine overdosing. Not too long ago a case was reported in Los Angeles involving three youngsters with behavior problems whose drug experiences sent them to the hospital. After taking an overdose of amphetamines, they all exhibited characteristic paranoid behavior for days following their use of the drugs. They mumbled incoherently and were plagued by intense anxieties that required immediate hospital treatment.

Another case was reported in New York concerning a fourteen-year-old girl who swallowed a number of amphetamine pills used by her mother for weight reduction. She lapsed into a psychosis during which she hallucinated and displayed violent behavior for weeks afterward. It was subsequently established that she had schizophrenic tendencies that had been accentuated by the drug.

The record of speed in the United States is not pretty. Besides the everyday misuse of amphetamine prescriptions, there are the speed freaks, the underground users of methedrine. Hippies have recently put out posters warning that "Speed Kills." By using the most potent of all amphetamines—methedrine—they have learned firsthand the dangers inherent in its indiscriminate use. Special clinics, such as the one in the Haight-Ashbury districts of San Francisco, have been established to treat the victims of "bum" acid and STP trips as well as to provide medical care for the undernourished, trembling bodies wasted by the effects of methedrine.

As a rule, there is little risk in taking amphetamine under a doctor's supervision. It has already been noted that the effects vary with the individual and the dosage. Nervousness, garrulousness and insomnia are side effects that, when accompanying minor doses, are not necessarily alarming. If, however, the dosages are increased over a period of time, the user may become easily agitated and his nervousness may progress into psychotic behavior. He may also suffer tremors and hallucinations, as well as digestive, respiratory, and circulatory troubles.

According to a California research team headed by Dr. John C. Kramer as quoted in the *Journal of the AMA*, injection of a drug such as methedrine (most amphetamines are taken orally) produces "a sudden generalized, overwhelming, pleasureful feeling called a 'flash' or a 'rush.' " Usually the need for action follows this flood of sensations. Sometimes the action is expressed in violence.

"You take some of those pills and you're ready to do anything," said one user. "You feel like you're superman. You're afraid of no one and intimidated by nothing."

According to another, the most pleasurable part is "the rush—an incredible feeling that your motor is running full speed. You actually believe you can accomplish anything. You feel you can demolish anything that stands in your way."

Others admit that extreme usage results in paranoiac episodes in which "you start believing cops are following you everywhere, that your telephone is tapped, and the mailman is keeping your letters from you."

Despite the hippie buttons proclaiming that "Speed Kills," tragic incidents involving amphetamines continue to occur. Extremely high doses of the drug have resulted in a number of deaths. A student at Purdue University collapsed in the midst of an exam, and a cyclist died during a European bike race. A report by John W. Rawlin of Southern Illinois University details the case of a thirty-six-year-old soldier who killed himself by taking large quantities of amphetamines. The autopsy revealed extensive brain damage. "The brain was removed with the hope of preserving it intact. But the tissues were so soft and crumbly that they collapsed before preservation could be attempted."

Because chronic methedrine users may become paranoid, suffer brain damage, or loss of memory, violence is not an uncommon occurrence. At the same time, to rub salt into the wounds of the speed freak, the quality of certain types of black-market methedrine engenders additional problems. Impure speed causes abscesses and swollen lips and eyes. Since the drug is injected intravenously, underground methedrine users also run the risk of contracting hepatitis from dirty needles. Although it is not physically addicting, methedrine hooks the user in a more subtle way; the worst part of the speed trip is coming down, and therefore the heavy user stops, sleeps, gets up, and shoots again, forever staving off the inevitable "crash."

"From descriptions of the intensity of the paranoid state and the hyperactivity associated with amphetamine use, crimes of violence by amphetamine users appear likely in the future," writes Dr. John Kramer in his study published in the *Journal of the AMA*.

The connection between amphetamines and crime is substantiated particularly by reports from abroad. The United States so far has been spared the serious amphetamine crime wave which became so alarming in Great Britain and Japan that medical authorities in those countries at one time considered banning the drug outright.

A striking example of the social malaise caused by unrestricted amphetamine use is illustrated by the "stimulant epidemic" that swept Japan in the late forties and early fifties. At its worst there were between half-a-million and a million habitual users who were responsible for a disproportionate amount of social unrest.

When the amphetamine-control laws went into effect in 1954, the number of arrests totaled fifty-five thousand violators. Between May and June of that year more than ten thousand persons were taken into custody, fifty-two percent of whom were found to be virtual addicts. In Great Britain, notes Dr. Connell, half of the sixty murders committed during a period of two months were by felons who "had some connection with amphetamine misuse."

The most recent crime to raise the hackles of authorities about amphetamine misuse in the United States concerned the "Linda and Groovy" case—two young speedheads who were found murdered in an East Village basement in New York City. Although speed did not figure in the work of the two suspected murderers apprehended later, the subsequent details of amphetamine misuse by the two victims shed a somber light on the hippie drug situation.

Some authorities insist that the connection between amphetamines and juvenile delinquency has been overestimated. The possibility that in a few individuals the drug may release latent antisocial behavior is not ruled out but, on the whole, they believe, amphetamines hold true to their reputation of promoting better adjustment to the social environment.

On the other hand, one of the chief reasons for police opposition to the wide circulation of the drugs concerns the fact that youngsters on amphetamines tend to stay up later than usual. This results in an increased potential for disturbances and unruly activities.

Detective Sergeant Howard addressing a symposium on drugs and delinquency in 1965 (reported in the *Medico-Legal Journal*) said: "It seems to me very theoretical to say that 'A' committed the theft because he had just taken pep pills. It is possible he would have committed the theft anyway and without the pills most probably would have made a better job of it, and maybe, with the associated bravado, would not have been caught."

It is the drug's *side effects*—insomnia, aggressiveness, anxiety, and touches of paranoia, especially with the come-down—that are likely to be the major force behind the crimes committed or attributed to amphetamine users.

Many a meth-head claims that methedrine increases the sex urge and enhances the pleasures of intercourse. The California study by Dr. John C. Kramer reported that in a group survey most of the subjects agreed that "sexual interest is enhanced considerably." Only two men of the group "indicated that their interest was diminished." Many assert that the drug delays orgasm and prolongs intercourse.

At the same time, other studies—such as Rawlin's at Southern Illinois University—show that, for the most part, the sexual motivations induced by amphetamines seem to turn off just as many users as they turn on. Some physicians, as a matter of fact, refuse to prescribe amphetamines for males with potency problems.

Again, in Dr. Kramer's study, repressed sexual deviance activated by the stimulus of amphetamines, especially the powerful methedrine, numbered only a few cases, which were subsequently rejected on the basis of insubstantial evidence.

D. S. Bell and W. H. Trethowan quote in the *Archives of General Psychiatry* a study they made in 1961 of thirteen amphetamine users who also displayed an extraordinary variety of sexual deviations. They noted that the factor of original personality disturbance in creating this condition was of prime importance in the use of the drug.

This study, carried out in Australia, revealed that among the subjects there were six cases with a family history of addiction to alcohol or drugs as well as a general record of mental illness in seven families. Of the thirteen only four had no history of prior trouble of this kind. Twelve out of the thirteen subjects had been openly rejected by their parents; the exception was an orphan brought up on an island by a stepfather who treated him cruelly.

Bell and Trethowan report the claims of one couple to the effect that with amphetamines they could prolong sexual intercourse to ten hours or more. The authors conclude, however, that in most cases the drug can increase sexual desire if it is already present, but actually reduces performance.

All patients said they used amphetamine because it made them feel powerful and self-possessed. On the other hand, the researchers stress that amphetamine indulgence—from the study recording the personalities of these people prior to drug use—invariably betrays "the presence of considerable personality defects." There are always two sides of a fence.

CHAPTER TWENTY-TWO

THE SPEED SCENE: THE LOGISTICS OF METH

Teen-Age Speed Freaks

In the 1950's, on a not particularly exciting weekend, the indulging teen-ager's ordinary dose of speed was probably equal to the weekly dose of thirty micrograms allowed soldiers in World War II. Under combat conditions the GI could draw on a supply of amphetamines—mainly benzedrine and dexedrine—of ten micrograms in twelve hours. In Vietnam at present, amphetamines are also used on a similar basis—in probably slightly larger amounts—but figures on dosage allowed the enlisted man are not yet available.

The teen-agers' thirty-milligram dose, although not a paltry amount, is only a quarter of the maximum dose recommended for benzedrine in certain clinical applications. The manufacturer of Drinamyl, for instance, recommends a dose of three pills per day, the last to be taken not after 4 P.M. because of the tendency to reduce sleep. Today, teen-agers out on a binge prefer to forego sleep rather than miss the weekend fun and tend to pop six to a dozen of these pills at one gulp. It is this disregard for caution in dosage consumed that poses the biggest problem in regard to amphetamine use.

Having seen their parents indulge in various mind-altering substances not considered taboo—from tranquilizers to sleeping pills—the youngsters' faith in anything pharmaceutical borders on the mystical. They seem to consider anything in pill form safe and beneficial, although this belief is especially ill-advised in the case of amphetamines.

In the United States today, it is this "speed scene" that has many parents and authorities worried. A growing percentage of the young users, bored or unaffected by the action of the pills, have graduated from oral doses (i.e., tablets or capsules) to injecting the drug intravenously. They have created an underground with rapidly growing territorial borders that strikingly parallels the world of the heroin addict. The staple of this speed culture is the fast-acting (almost instant) methedrine.

The methedrine, sold in crystalline form in small envelopes, even looks like heroin and is being used in much the same way. The white powder ("crystal") is mixed with a few drops of water in a spoon until it has dissolved. In the case of adulterated methedrine, which is brown or gray in appearance and dotted with black spots, the substance is "cooked" in a manner similar to the procedure for cooking heroin. Like the junkie of yesteryear, the meth-head uses paraphernalia (called "works") with which he "shoots up" by employing an eyedropper instead of the complete hypodermic needle apparatus common for injections.

Those who "shoot" the drug in this way, rather than take it in pill form, follow the junkie method of raising a vein in the lower arm or, if this proves impossible, proceed to inject the methedrine into the wrist, hands, legs, and even shoulders and back. The meth-head prefers shooting the drug in order to get the euphoric flash (the rush of the injection's instantaneous effect).

Underground laboratories are today churning out methedrine for thirty dollars a pound, which street dealers will eventually sell for twenty-five dollars a gram. Not surprisingly, the illegal manufacture of speed has developed into one of the biggest rackets since heroin. The market has evolved from what was once a minor sideline of pot pushers and other drug dealers, unscrupulous pharmacists and physicians—known as "scriptwriters"—who dealt mainly in oral doses of the earlier amphetamines, benzedrine and dexedrine.

Enough amphetamines to supply every man, woman, and child in the United States with forty-six doses leave the premises of the thousands of drug manufacturers each year to start their journey to legitimate and illegitimate markets alike.

It is estimated that close to one-half of these billions of doses ultimately find their way onto the black market every year; and this does not include the product of the hundreds of illegal underground drug manufacturers. More than fifty million prescriptions for amphetamines were filled in this country in 1967 alone. At the same time, experts project that at least another half-million persons use amphetamines annually without ever seeing a doctor, or a prescription.

The business resulting from this extra-legal enterprise underwrites a half-billion-dollar traffic in the drug every year. The Bureau of Drug Abuse Control and now its successor, the Bureau of Narcotics and Dangerous Drugs (BNDD), which was established in 1968, stands virtually powerless in the face of such a staggering volume of violations; it still spends half its time on "accountability" surveys at commercial drug houses. The bureau's agents concentrate especially on the "fly-by-night" houses—drug manufacturers whose orientation is especially designed to take advantage of the underground market where they can sell their wares—amphetamines, tranquilizers, and barbiturates—at a price higher than the regular wholesale price they would ordinarily receive from druggists and doctors.

The pills (in strengths mainly of five to ten milligrams) cost about one to two pennies each when purchased on prescription at a drugstore. On the black market, however, the price per pill, usually benzedrine and dexedrine, runs from two for twenty-five cents to one dollar each, depending on the circumstances. The price for methedrine is higher.

Another thriving source for the black market is the supply of amphetamines pilfered from the production lines of the firms that manufacture the drug. A supply is also smuggled or imported illegally into this country from Europe, Japan, Taiwan, and Hong Kong. This total is supplemented by a variety of domestically produced underground methedrine.

Although the Mafia controls the heroin distribution in this country, the black market in amphetamines is similar to that of the hallucinogens in that there is no hierarchy of criminal drug interests running its operations. A few loosely based crime groups have a tenuous hold on the underground amphetamine channels, but a good percentage of the illicit sales are the province of amateurs.

Just how loose and inefficient the government controls on the drug manufacturer are was illustrated in 1965 by a New York television newsman. As part of a special program dealing with the underground drug world, the newsman, using a phony letterhead in his correspondence with fifty ethical drug companies, ordered a supply of amphetamines and barbiturates. Twenty of the companies contacted answered his request and gladly filled the orders for close to one million tablets. The newsman paid a little more than six hundred dollars for this supply—a price that would have been agreeable to any wholesaler; as a middleman he could have sold his inventory on the drugstore market for $54,000. Its black-market value was in excess of a half-million dollars.

Another black-market source of amphetamines are doctors and pharmacists. On one level, hippies with weight problems can readily cop amphetamines if they can convince their physician to give them a prescription for the drug as part of a reducing program. For this very reason, fat hippies are sometimes popular among their group as a ready source for the drug. Although most doctors and druggists do not willingly involve themselves in this type of enterprise, there are some who find it difficult to resist the huge profits to be made in dealing in these pills. Because they can obtain supplies from drug manufacturers for a fraction of a penny per pill and sell them for twenty-five cents each or more, there are a small number of "scriptwriters" in the medical profession who readily take advantage of this high profit rate. The Bureau of Drug Abuse Control reported that in a ten-year period up until 1967 better than a thousand druggists and doctors were tried for malpractice in dispensing these drugs too liberally.

The World Health Organization and the UN Commission on Narcotic Drugs have also discovered flagrant violations by drug companies around the world in the dispensing of amphetamines. Some countries in Europe and in the Far East where the drugs are not as strictly controlled as they are in the United States were doing a flourishing business. Drug smugglers and importers would bring the drugs into this country in powder form under false labels and then proceed to package the powder in either capsules or pills that were destined for black-market distribution.

From Italy, shipments of illegal methedrine are known to have reached this country via the Mafia connections in Montreal and Toronto in Canada. Although international organizations, such as the World Health Organization, have tried to impose tighter controls on the distribution of the amphetamines, the limitations of the enforcing agencies remain a problem and the illicit distribution of drugs continues to flourish.

The federal agency first responsible for imposing restrictions and attempting to enforce them for the amphetamines as well as for the hallucinogens was the Bureau of Drug Abuse Control (BDAC), now absorbed in the Bureau of Narcotics and Dangerous Drugs. The BDAC was established in 1966 when such drugs as LSD, speed, DMC, DET, STP, and other hallucinogens were placed under its control.

Despite the fact that they seize thousands of bootleg pills each year, the agents admit being nowhere close to stopping the illicit traffic. They point out that they are now dealing with a new breed of underground drug dealer—not at all like the old-time heroin dealer with connections to the Mafia.

A good many of the underground manufacturers—usually chemists with few scruples just out of college—see in illicit drug production an easy way of making a quick fortune. Using their knowledge to set up underground labs, they usually operate in conjunction with other partners to establish a huge distribution system—very much like a modern corporation. Unlike the heroin-distribution organization that uses professional chemists in overseas countries, such as France and North Africa, for the processing of the drug, the new drug dealers for amphetamines and the hallucinogens manufacture their product from start to finish without outside encumbrances.

One of this "new breed of drug dealer" was recently apprehended by Bureau of Drug Abuse Control agents in a raid on an underground lab in New York City. They found that the student chemist had photocopied data referring to the manufacture of DMT from a biochemistry textbook in the library of the school of graduate studies at Columbia University.

One large-scale methedrine supplier had an organization that included four huge laboratories and an elaborate group of underground drug retailers for distribution of his product to both campus and hippie communities. The people involved in this type of enterprise are simply in it for the money, netting as much as $50,000 to $100,000 a year—and that tax-free.

To produce methedrine, the underground chemist must first obtain the raw material—phenyl-2-propanone. It is obtained from such sources as contacts working in legal drug manufacturing plants, hospitals, or from the various overseas countries where it may be purchased legally and then shipped either by mail or hand carried to this country.

Many of these underground entrepreneurs began as marijuana pushers in college. As the market for methedrine began to expand, however, they switched to distributing amphetamine as a more profitable line. Compared to marijuana, the manufacture of amphetamine shows a series of distinct advantages. Marijuana must be smuggled into this country and it is bulky to ship. Also, its present distribution system is flooded by thousands of small-time operators contributing to a prevailing chaos that is difficult to control. Furthermore, dealing in pot is a felony, while amphetamine distribution and sale is only a misdemeanor. In addition, it was found that amphetamine can be manufactured at a much lower cost than that involved in the purchase and smuggling of marijuana into this country from Mexico.

Previous sellers of marijuana introduced their customers to the new drug on the street and on campus. The campus market, however, remained relatively small since most college students—aware of the dangers of speed—prefer marijuana. Amphetamine manufacturers found their biggest market among the teen-agers and hippies who were supplied mainly by off-campus marijuana dealers.

It was not until the hippie boom of 1966-67 that the amphetamines came into real popularity and the market suddenly opened up. Today the East Coast alone uses hundreds of pounds of methedrine each week. As the underground drug dealers found that amphetamine was a seller's market with demand outweighing the supply, they revved up the production line accordingly.

Going down the scale of the amphetamine-drug distributors, the street dealer who buys from the illicit manufacturer and distributor usually purchases the methedrine in ounces and sells it in "spoons." Most of the small-time pushers, by purchasing a half-ounce at $100 or a full ounce at $200, can make a handsome profit by selling "spoons" for approximately $20 each. Thus, for an outlay of $100 for a half-ounce they can sell approximately fifteen "spoons" resulting in a gross of $300 and a net profit of $200 over their investment.

Thus, the drug which the illicit drug entrepreneur manufactures for $30 a pound realizes better than $10,000 a pound when it is eventually distributed on the underground market.

The above method of distribution is followed by the small-time street dealer of meth who is usually hooked on the drug. By pushing methedrine he can make enough money to pay expenses and keep himself supplied with the drug for his own use. Usually he is not physically addicted, but is so psychologically hung-up on the drug he cannot do without it. Although the name "speed freak" is applied to many hippies who use the drug in small amounts, the people truly deserving of this nomenclature are those types who use the drug constantly and over long periods.

The true speed freak's entire life is built around the white crystals of methedrine. A whole new mystique has formed around this drug—a mystique that has much more in common with that surrounding heroin than the myths that envelop LSD and pot. Like the heroin user of the 1930's who despairingly turned from the reality of the Depression scene and the hopelessness he felt about his existence, the young users of methedrine are likewise a social phenomenon. College students, less alienated and more informed about the effects and dangers of the various drugs, continue to shy away from the amphetamines—preferring to use pot and acid.

The big market for speed seems to be in the growing hippie and suburban teen-age market. It is these youngsters, the disaffected from the hippie ghettoes and the bored and alienated youth from the bleak suburbs who develop into speed freaks and become completely tied up in the mystique of the drug. The Bureau of Narcotics and Dangerous Drugs estimated that more youngsters under eighteen are now using speed than LSD. They spend hours trying to buy the drug from underground connections, and from the time they find a dealer to the moment they shoot the drug into their veins, they become trapped in the speed scene—an unsavory part of the overall drug environment that has become so deeply rooted in our mass culture.

AFTERWORD

by Stanley Krippner, Ph.D.

Each new discovery is potentially destructive as well as progressive. The discovery of the New World brought about the slave trade and the destruction of the American Indians as well as the expansion of knowledge and trade. The development of gunpowder facilitated man's mastery of nature but also made possible the widespread military infliction of pain and misery. The invention of the cotton gin proved to be an economic boon but helped perpetuate slavery. Self-propelled land and air vehicles are as valuable during times of war as they are during times of peace. Atomic energy may eventually assist industrial progress but, in the meantime, has emerged as a specter of death and destruction.

With the advent of psychochemistry, it was inevitable that consciousness-altering drugs would be discovered and produced. It was probably just as inevitable that the new chemicals, despite their considerable utility in research and psychotherapy, would fall into illegal usage and produce blown minds and wasted lives.

In this book, Allen Geller and Maxwell Boas have painted a vivid picture of these psychochemicals—presenting the full spectrum of delights and dangers inherent in their use. They have done an especially fine job of introducing their readers to the horrors of amphetamine abuse. It is apparent to me that methedrine (an unusually powerful amphetamine) is the most dangerous drug now on the black market—a drug which often leaves a trail of irreversibly brain-injured addicts and potentially homicidal psychotics in its wake. Geller and Boas portray the frustration faced by federal agencies in combating amphetamine abuse.

In my opinion, education provides a better approach than prosecution in preventing abuse of amphetamines and other potentially dangerous drugs. I have found that rational educational programs are of the most help—programs in which students are presented with the facts and allowed to make their own decisions. A national student-directed educational program is now in operation, directed by the Student Association for the Study of Hallucinogens (with headquarters at Beloit College, Beloit, Wisconsin).

A rational educational program will also demonstrate the value of LSD—when administered by a competent guide in pleasant surroundings—and the potential harm it can do when taken informally using black market supplies. My colleagues and I have discovered black-market LSD which contains methedrine, heroin, atropine, and strychnine—and some which contains no LSD at all.

It is possible that these impurities present physiological as well as psychological hazards; no healthy human subject taking pharmaceutical LSD has yet been found with broken chromosomes, including several dozen infants born to women who ingested LSD during pregnancy. On the other hand, chromosomal breaks have been noticed in many black-market LSD users, as well as among some of their babies. I, personally, have long argued for the establishment of college research centers that would allow all interested students who pass basic screening tests to have a legal, well-guided LSD, mescaline, or psilocybin experience with chemically pure, pharmaceutical substances. There is no law or statute that would prevent a university clinic from making immediate application for the establishment of such a program to the National Institute of Mental Health. If several colleges were to make applications, the requests could not be ignored or continually rejected.

In the meantime, educational campaigns are needed to inform people as to the risks involved in ingesting black-market LSD. Unfortunately, many of the current educational campaigns are doomed to fail because they include marijuana among the "dangerous drugs" in their curriculum. Any amount of positive value which may result from informing students as to the dangers of heroin, glue-sniffing, methedrine, depressants, and black-market LSD will fail to materialize if misinformation about marijuana is presented.

Intelligent youngsters need only to spot one flaw in an anti-marijuana diatribe to entertain serious suspicions about the validity of the entire presentation. The lament, "They lied to us about marijuana, perhaps they're lying to us about LSD," has become commonplace. It also arouses suspicion whenever alcohol and tobacco are *not* included in the list of "dangerous drugs"; many students began to suspect that the program's main concern is the maintenance of the established legal-social order rather than the health and well-being of the young.

In 1968, on behalf of an *ad hoc* committee, I wrote to the U.S. Attorney General and to other government officials urging a massive research program on the effects of marijuana. If the hazards of marijuana usage were found to be minimal, we urged a regulatory process under which a legal outlet could be provided for the substance. In the meantime we suggested a moratorium on imprisonments for marijuana users, suggesting educational and psychiatric alternatives for offenders.

Since the letter was written, a number of research studies have been published, among them a paper in *Science* (May 16, 1969) disclosing that the driving ability of marijuana users is not impaired while they are under the substance's influence (alcohol, on the other hand, caused them to make significantly more driving errors). A spokesman for the National Institute of Mental Health recently stated that, to date, no evidence has been produced indicating that short-term marijuana use is harmful. Dr. Philip Handler, chairman of the National Science Board, stated (on June 7, 1969) that there is no evidence linking marijuana usage to stronger drugs and no evidence that marijuana itself is addictive.

The U.S. Supreme Court has declared unconstitutional key provisions of the federal anti-marijuana legislation—yet marijuana arrests continue to rise as law enforcement officers struggle desperately to stem the tide of this significant social change. My own survey which indicated that 50 percent of American troops in Vietnam use marijuana was confirmed in 1969 by Dr. John Talbott after spending twelve months with a psychiatric team there. When these troops—and their newly discovered interest—return to the United States, the conflict with the legal establishment cannot help but intensify.

I personally know hundreds of persons of all ages who smoke marijuana. Of these, two individuals have had unpleasant, psychotic-like reactions and, in my opinion, should not try the substance again. A few others use marijuana several times a day and seem to have suffered a deterioration in judgment and problem-solving abilities. The others, as I have observed them, have not been affected adversely. Indeed, some have changed for the better, becoming more interested in art, in politics, in religion, and showing greater productivity in their work and a heightened capacity to relate to other people. Nevertheless, for some people there may be deleterous effects to marijuana usage.

Yet, no matter what negative effects of marijuana use there may prove to be, it is inconceivable that they should match the blatant wickedness and evil currently resulting from the outdated anti-marijuana laws and their enforcement. A friend of mine who teaches in a well-known university was recently falsely accused of selling marijuana to a narcotics officer who masqueraded as a student and attended the professor's class. Despite the fact that the professor produced witnesses testifying that he was at a social gathering when the marijuana sale allegedly took place, he was convicted and sentenced to a lengthy prison term (which he is currently appealing). The narcotics officer was given a promotion and a raise in pay despite the fact that the transcript of the case shows glaring inconsistencies in his testimony.

An artist friend was recently approached by an "art dealer" who promised to buy three of his paintings, but only if the artist would secure some marijuana for him. The artist complied, even though he does not smoke marijuana or use any other drug. Upon delivery of the paintings and the marijuana, the artist was arrested by the "art dealer" who proved to be an undercover narcotics officer.

An actor friend was recently visited by a vacationing college student who had known his family for fifteen years. Shortly after the actor and the student smoked marijuana together, the actor was arrested. It developed that the student had been apprehended on marijuana charges by the narcotics squad at his school. He had been promised immunity if he would serve as an "informer" and was sent to infiltrate the home of his artist friend.

Here, then, we come face to face with the negative aspects of marijuana use. The wickedness is in the laws and regulations that can bring out the very worst traits of the twisted individuals who sometimes enter the law-enforcement field. The evil is in the enforcement policies that can so corrupt a young man's integrity that he takes advantage of a personal friend to untangle himself from his own legal difficulties.

In these days of agonizing wars, racial conflicts, and poverty problems, we need all the fine minds and dedicated spirits we can muster if civilization is to survive and progress. One justified source of alienation is the power establishment's unjust and unreasonable response to exploration with psychedelic plants and the new psychochemicals. If repression is not replaced by education, and if intolerance is not replaced by understanding, our hopes for the future and our vision of the human potential will be gravely jeopardized. The "drug beat" in its present form, perhaps, is an immature but significant precursor of a new type of consciousness emerging in our time—an expanded awareness stressing man's commitment to love, beauty, joy, and truth.

If the positive aspects of it are supported and nurtured, the negative aspects can be handled by education rather than by repression. Finally, mankind can progress and go about its business, having rationally and wisely handled the results of yet another new invention and discovery.

Stanley Krippner, Ph.D., is Director, Dream Laboratory, Maimonides Medical Center, New York City; Lecturer in Special Education, Graduate School, Wagner College; and Director of Research, New York Institute for the Achievement of Human Potential. He is also a Fellow in the American Society of Clinical Hypnosis, and serves on the Advisory Board of the Student Association for the Study of Hallucinogens.

BIBLIOGRAPHY

ABRAMSON, Harold, ed. *The Use of LSD in Psychotherapy and Alcoholism.* Indianapolis: Bobbs-Merrill, 1967.

ALLENTUCK, S., and BOWMAN, K. "The Psychiatric Aspects of Marihuana Intoxication." *American Journal of Psychiatry* 99 (1942).

ALPERT, R., COHEN, S., and SCHILLER, L. *LSD.* New York: New American Library, 1966.

BAUDELAIRE, Charles. *Les Paradis Artificiels.* Translated by R. Symons. London: The Casanova Society of London, 1925.

BISCHOFF, W.H. *The Ecstacy Drugs.* Delray Beach: University Circle Press, 1966.

BISHOP, M.G. *The Discovery of Love.* New York: Dodd, Mead & Company, 1963.

BLUM, Richard. *Utopiates: The Use and Users of LSD-25.* New York: Atherton Press, 1965.

BROWN, David. *The Milder Hallucinogens: Nutmeg, Morning Glory Seeds, Marihuana.* London: Westmount Press, 1965.

BROWN, T.T. *The Enigma of Drug Addiction.* Springfield, Ill.: Charles C. Thomas, 1961.

BURROUGHS, William. *Junkie.* New York: Ace Books, 1953.

BURROUGHS, William, and GINSBURG, Allen. *The Yage Letters.* San Francisco: City Lights Books, 1963.

CHARBONNEAU, L. *Psychedelic-40.* New York: Bantam Books, 1965.

CHAREN, S., and PERELMAN, L. "Personality Studies of Marihuana Addicts," *American Journal of Psychiatry* 102, no. 5 (March, 1946).

CHOLDEN, Louis, ed. *Lysergic Acid Diethylamide and Mescaline in Experimental Psychiatry.* New York: Grune and Stratton, 1956.

CHOPRA, R.N., and G.S. *The Present Position of Hemp Drug Addiction in India.* India: Indian Medical Research, Thacker, Spink, 1939.

CHOPRA, R.N., G.S., and I.C. "Cannabis Sativa in Relation to Mental Diseases and Crime in India," *Indian Journal of Medical Research* 30, no. 1.

COHEN, Sidney. *The Beyond Within.* New York: Atheneum, 1964.

DeROPP, Robert S. *Drugs and the Mind.* New York: St. Martin's Press, 1957.

DODGE, C.R. *A Report on the Culture of Hemp and Jute in the United States.* Washington, D.C.: Government Printing Office, 1896.

———. *A Report on the Culture of Hemp and Jute in Europe.* Washington, D.C.: Government Printing Office, 1898.

DUNLAP, Jane. *Exploring Inner Space.* New York: Harcourt, Brace & World, 1961.

EBIN, David, ed. *The Drug Experience.* New York: Orion Press, 1961.

HECTOR, France. *Musk, Hashish and Blood.* New York: Falstaff.

GAUTIER, T. *Le Club des Hachischins.* Paris: Feuilleton de la Presse Medicale, 1843.

GOLDSTEIN, R. *1 in 7: Drugs on Campus.* New York: Walker and Company, 1966.

HOFFER, Abram. "D-Lysergic Acid Diethylamide (LSD): A Review of its Present Status." *Clinical Pharmacology and Therapeutics* March-April, 1965.

HUXLEY, Aldous. *Island.* New York: Harper & Row, 1962.

———. *The Doors of Perception.* New York: Harper & Row, 1954.

LEARY, Timothy. *Psychedelic Prayers.* Kerhonkson, New York: Poets Press, 1966.

LEARY, Timothy; METZNER, Ralph; and WEIL, G.M., eds. *The Psychedelic Reader.* New York: University Books, 1965.

LEARY, Timothy; METZNER, Ralph; and ALPERT, Richard, eds. *The Psychedelic Experience.* New York: University Books, 1964.

LINDESMITH, A.E. *The Addict and the Law.* Bloomington: Indiana University Press, 1965.

LJUBISA, Grlic. "Recent Advances in the Chemical Research of Cannabis," *Bulletin on Narcotics* 16, no. 4.

LUDLOW, Fitz Hugh. *The Hasheesh Eater.* New York: Harper & Brothers, 1857.

MASTERS, R.E.L., and HOUSTON, Jean. *The Varieties of Psychedelic Experience.* New York: Holt, Rinehart and Winston, 1966.

MAUER, D.W., and VOGEL, V.H. *Narcotics and Narcotics Addiction.* Springfield, Ill.: Charles C. Thomas, 1962.

Mayor's Committee on Marihuana. *The Marihuana Problem in the City of New York.* Tempe, Arizona: Jaques Cattell Press, 1944.

McCLURE, Michael. *Meat Science Essays.* San Francisco: City Lights Books, 1963.

MEZZROW, Mess. *Really the Blues.* New York: New American Library, 1964.

NEWLAND, Constance A. *My Self and I.* New York: Coward-McCann, 1962.

ROSEMAN, Bernard. *LSD: The Age of Mind.* Hollywood: Wilshire Book Company, 1963.

SCARLINGELLI, F. "Spectrophotometric Identification of Marihuana," *Journal of Association of Official Agricultural Chemists* 44, no. 2 (1961).

SHUR, Edwin. *Narcotics Addiction in Britain and America.* Bloomington: Indiana University Press, 1962.

SILER, J.F. "Marihuana Smoking in Panama," *The Military Surgeon* 73, no. 5 (1933).

SOLOMON, David. *The Marihuana Papers.* Indianapolis: Bobbs-Merrill, 1966.

———. ed. *LSD: The Consciousness-Expanding Drug.* New York: G. P. Putnam's Sons, 1964.

TAYLOR, Norman. *Narcotics: Nature's Dangerous Gifts.* New York: Dell, 1963.

TOMKINS, W. F., and ANSLINGER, H. *The Traffic in Narcotics.* New York: Funk & Wagnalls, 1953.

WALTON, R.P. *Marihuana: America's New Drug Problem.* Philadelphia: Lippincott, 1938.

WATTS, Alan W. *The Joyous Cosmology.* New York: Pantheon Books, 1962.

White House Conference on Narcotics and Drug Abuse: September, 1962. Washington, D.C.: Government Printing Office, 1963.

WILLIAMS, E.G. "Studies on Marihuana and Pyrhexyl Compound," *Public Health Reports* no. 61 (1946).

WOLFF. Pablo. *Marihuana in Latin America.* Washington, D.C.: Linacre Press, 1949.

ZAHCROUPER. Howard. *The Psychology of the Drug User.* Diller Press, 1959.

INDEX

Ad Hoc Panel on Drug Abuse, The, 97-98
Adams, Dr. Roger, 41
Aerosol sprays, 236-237
Africa, 4, 5, 7, 13, 28, 35, 36, 37, 38, 40, 73, 82, 103, 260
Alcohol, xi, xii, 5, 56, 65, 66, 74, 79-80, 96, 103-109, 112-114, 118, 170, 172, 200, 233, 249
Alcoholics, 90, 196, 221-224, 233
Alcoholics Anonymous, 222, 223
Algeria, 7, 13
Allentuck, Dr. Samuel, 103
Alpert, Dr. Richard, 163-166, 176, 191, 226
American Medical Association, 88
American Medical Association Drug Committee, 244
American Psychiatric Association, 98
Amphetamine Psychosis (Connell), 249
Amphetamines, ix, xiii, xiv, 54, 92, 151-152, 190, 194, 233-262
  abuse of, 233-238
  addiction, 248-249, 252-253
  sex and, 255
  U.S., 233-238, 251-254, 256-262
Amylnitrite, 235-236
Anaphrodisiacs, 225
Anslinger, Harry J., 26, 116, 117, 119
Aphrodisiacs, 102-104, 225, 228
Appetite suppression, 244-245
Arabian Nights, 6, 17, 102
Arabs, 6-7
Archives of General Psychiatry, 254-255
Army alpha test, 49
Artificial Paradise, The (Baudelaire), 8-13
Asia, 3, 4, 5, 34, 82
Ascorbic acid, 195
Association of Military Surgeons of the United States, 147
Australia, 255
Autistic children, 218
Aztecs, 13-14

Banana peels, smoking, 236
Barbiturates, 233, 234, 241, 249
Baudelaire, Charles, 7, 8-13, 43, 57
Beatles, 31, 63
Becker, Dr. Howard S., 33, 96, 101-102
Bell, D. S., 248-249, 254-255
Belladonna, 235-236
Bellevue adult-intelligence test, 49
Bender, Dr. Lauretta M., 218
Benji, 6
Benzedrine, 54, 233, 234, 244, 256
  cost of, 258
Bergess, Richard, 124
Bhang, 3, 4, 5, 38, 39, 73, 86, 102
Binet line-suggestibility test, 50
Birth defects, 91, 185-186
Blackburn, J. M., 241
Blum, Dr. Richard, 104
Bono, Victor, 134
Boston Herald, 165
Boston University Medical Center, 43, 54-57, 60
Bowman, Dr. Karl, 103
Brazil, 117
British Columbia, 223
Bromberg, Dr. Walter, 87-88, 98-99, 173
Bromide, 249
Brown, Thorvald T., 103
Bruce, Lenny, xi
Buckman, John, 229-230
Bulletin of Narcotics, 100
Bureau of Drug Abuse Control (BDAC), 179, 185, 258, 259, 260
Bureau of Narcotics, 3, 25, 26, 33, 36, 37, 42, 55, 80, 83, 89, 95, 115-117, 123, 129-132, 151, 185
  establishment of, 115
Bureau of Narcotics and Dangerous Drugs (BNDD), 185, 258, 260, 262
Burma, 149
Burr, C. W., 102
Burrell, Dr. Craig, 182
Burroughs, William, 29-30, 59
Burton, Richard, 102

Caffeine, 108, 112
California Bureau of Narcotic Enforcement, 97
Cambodia, 149, 150
Canada, 40, 222-224, 259
Cancellation test, 49
Cannabinaceae, 53

Cannabis, 3, 4, 5, 22-23, 24
Cannabis Americana, 53
"Cannabis Habit, The: A Review of Recent Psychiatric Literature" (Murphy), 100, 109
Cannabis Indica, 53
Cannabis sativa, 3
Cannabis sativa L, 34-42, 147
Cannabis Sinensis, 53
Caribbean Islands, 129, 136
Carson, Johnny, 30
Carstairs, G. M., 108-109
Castalia Foundation, 167-169
Charas, 39-40
Children, autistic, 218-219
Chillum (pipe), 67
China, 3-4, 53
Chopra, Dr. G. S., 85, 86, 102, 405
Chopra, Dr. R. N., 4-5, 85, 86, 102
Ciba Symposia, 82
Claviceps purpurea, 156
Club des Hachischins, 7, 8, 11, 13, 18
Cocaine, 26, 60, 92
Cocktail method, 72
Codeine, 83, 235
Cohen, Dr. Sidney, 219, 226
Collins, Judy, 108
Collins dynamometer, 48
Commission of Psychochemical Education, 176
Committee to Legalize Marijuana (LeMar), 32, 125
"Concerning Cannabis Indica" (Robinson), 82
Confessions of an Opium Eater, The (De Quincey), 17-22
Connally, Judge Ben, 168
Connell, Dr. Philip H., 249-250, 253
Cooper, Florence, 172-173
Copping, 68-69
Cornell University Medical College, 53
Creativity, 76-77
Crime, 95-111, 128-144, 181, 258, 259, 260
Crime and Personality (Eysenck), 241, 243
"Cultural Factors in Choice of Intoxicants" (Carstairs), 108-109
"Curious Story Behind the New Cary Grant, The" (magazine article), 220
Customs, 132
Czechoslovakia, 40
Dagga, 38, 98
Daniel, Price, 116
Dawamesk, 7-8
De Quincey, Thomas, 17-22
Delirium tremens, 244
Delson, Judith M., 55
Delysid, 216
Department of Agriculture, 37
DET, 260
Dexedrine, 240, 256
  cost, 258
Dextro-amphetamine sulphate, 240
Dick, Fred, 89
Dimethyl-tryptamine (DMT), 175, 237-238, 260
DMC, 260
Doors of Perception (Huxley), 163, 242
Downey will-and-temperament test, 50
Drake, Betsy, 220
Drill, 183
Drinamyl, 256
Drug Abuse Control Amendment Act, 174, 177
Drug addiction, 56-58, 87-91, 248-249, 252-253
Drug habit, 87
Drug tolerance, 87
Duquenois test, 42
Dylan, Bob, ix

Egypt, 7, 112, 117
Eisenhower, Dwight D., 89
Emerick, Chester, 129
Enigma of Drug Addiction, The (Brown), 103
Esquire (magazine), 140-141
Expert Committee on Addiction-Producing Drugs, 117
Eysenck, H. J., 241, 243

Facelle, T. A., 89
Farmers' Bulletin, 37
Federal Bureau of Investigation, 18
Feinglass, Dr. Sanford, 100
Fetishism, 230
Fonteyn, Dame Margot, 31
Food, marijuana in, 72-73
Food and Drug Administration, 18, 31, 63, 79-80, 174-176, 178, 179, 182, 183, 237, 240, 245
Fort, Dr. Joel, 106-107
Forum board test, 49

Fox, Dr. James M., 80
France, 7-13, 24, 71, 112, 260
France, Hector, 102
Freon-12, 237
Freud, Sigmund, 218, 241-242
Friedenberg, E. Z., 108
Friedman, 84
Frigidity, 228-230
Frustration test, 50
Fulbright, William, 117

Galton whistle, 48-49
Ganja, 3, 38-39, 44, 54
Garawash, 73
Gautier, Théophile, 7, 13, 43
Geber, Dr. William F., 91, 94
Germany, 40, 158
Ginsberg, Allen, 29-30
Giordano, Henry L., 33, 89-90, 95, 100, 118
Glossary, xvi-xxiii
Goddard, Dr. James L., xii, 31, 63, 79-80
Gollan, Antoni, 31, 125-127
Gomila, Dr. Frank R., 24, 97
Goodenough test, 50
Grant, Cary, 220
Great Britain, 15, 63, 71, 93, 246-247, 249, 253
Greece, 4

Hallucinogens, xii, xiii, 42, 57-59, 92, 110, 122, 162, 169
  See also names of hallucinogens
Harrison Narcotics Act of 1922, 113-114
Hartman, Dr. Mortimer, 220
Harvard Alumni Bulletin (1967), 90
Harvard Crimson, 164, 165
Harvard Review, 166
Harvard University, 161-166
Hasan-I-Sabbah, 5-6
Hasheesh, 40, 44
Hasheesh Eater, The: Being Passages from the Life of a Pythagorean (Ludlow), 17
Hashheads, 67
Hashish, 3, 6, 22, 53, 54, 67, 102, 117
Hawaiian woodflowers, 236
Health, Education, and Welfare Department, 127
Heilman, John, 168
Hemp, 15-16, 35
Herodotus, 4
Heroin, 26, 42, 60, 64, 118, 120, 179, 235
  marijuana and, 79-94
Hippies, 62, 71, 73, 109, 129, 182-183, 184, 236, 237, 247, 251, 259, 261, 262
History of the Hemp Industry in Kentucky, A (Hopkins), 15
Hoffer, Dr. Abram, 218, 222
Hoffman, Dr. Albert, 155-158
Hoffman, Martin, 80
Holland, 15
Homosexuals, 84, 226, 230
Hong Kong, 258
Hopkins, James F., 15
Hornor, Boyd, 124
Houston, Dr. J., xii-xiv, 190-191, 192-193, 200, 201, 230
Howard, Sergeant, 254
Huxley, Aldous, 163, 164, 242

I Ching, x
"In The Marketplace of Free Ideas: A Look at the Passage of the Marijuana Tax Act" (Oteri and Silvergate), 126-127
India, 3, 4, 5, 14, 35-36, 37, 38-39, 44, 53, 54, 67, 73, 82, 85-86, 102, 108-109
Indian hemp plant, 3
Internal Revenue Department, 119
International Foundation for Internal Freedom (IFIF), 165, 167
International Narcotic Association, 25
International Narcotic Education Association, 25-26
Interstate Narcotic Association, 24-25
Italy, 40, 259

Japan, 16, 253, 258
Javits, Jacob, 118
Jazz world, 29, 30, 63, 120, 123
Johnson, Lyndon B., 89, 174, 177
Jonathan Winters Show (TV), 30
Journal of the American Medical Association, 81, 83, 88, 98, 252, 253
Journal of Nervous and Mental Diseases, 249

Kelman, Dr. Herbert, 165
Keniston, Kenneth, 32-33
Kerouac, Jack, 29-30

Kessler, Steven, 172-173
Kif, 3, 38, 44
Klee, Dr. Gerald, 171
Kohs block-design test, 49
Korean War, 147
Kramer, Dr. John C., 252, 253, 254
Kwalwasser-Dykema music tests, 48

La Guardia, Fiorello, 27-28, 44, 45
La Guardia Report, 27-28, 36, 41, 42-54, 58-60, 70, 73-75, 83-87, 89, 97, 99, 104, 107, 134, 137-138
Lancet, 241
Laos, 149, 150
Larick, George P., 245
Latin America, 13, 14, 28, 37, 82
Leary, Susan, 119
Leary, Dr. Timothy, xii; 10, 46, 75, 119, 157, 161-172, 175, 176, 187-188, 190, 191, 195, 203, 225
LeMar (organization), 32, 125
Level-of-aspiration test, 50
Librium, 194, 195
Liebert, Dr. Robert S., 61
Lindesmith, Dr. Alfred R., 90, 105-106, 116, 120-121
Ling, Dr. Thomas, 229-230
Linnaeus, Carolus, 34
Loeb, Dr. Howard A., 160
Lohman, Joseph, 122-123
London Evening Standard, 246
Loof-Bourrow personal-index test, 50
Look (magazine), 220
Louria, Dr. Donald, 32, 61, 93
Lowe, Dr. S., 44-45
LSD, x, xii-xiv, 8, 11, 12, 42, 46, 57-60, 62, 91, 92, 122, 155-230, 260
  compared legally to marijuana, 122
  congenial atmosphere for, 75-76
  death from, 159-160
  dosage, 195-196, 197
  the first trip, 155-160
  the impact of, 197-202
  measurement of, 194
  mental health and, 214-224
  set and setting, 187-190
  sex and, 200, 225-230
  smuggling of, 178
  U.S., 158-160, 178-186
  antilegislation, 171-177
    the Leary-Alpert complex, 161-170
    number of users, 180
  workings of, 187-196
LSD (Alpert and Cohen), 226
Ludlow, Fitz Hugh, 17-22, 43
Lysergic acid dyethylamide, *see* LSD

McClelland, Dr. David, 162, 166
McGlothlin, Dr. William, 57, 110-111
McLuhan, Marshall, 31
Mafia, 128, 131, 134, 181, 258, 259, 260
Magazines, 31, 32-33, 63, 85
Majum, 39, 73
Mandell, Dr. Arnold T., 246
Mansfield, Mike, 119
Manzul, 73
Marco Polo, 5, 6, 97
Marihuana, 38
"Marihuana or Indian Hemp and Its Preparations" (pamphlet), 25-26
Marihuana Problem in the City of New York (La Guardia Report), 27-28, 44-54
Marijuana, ix, xi-xii, xiii, 3-152, 190, 193, 261
  as an aphrodisiac, 102-104
  the authorities and, 112-127
  compared legally to LSD, 122
  congenial atmosphere for, 75-76
  cost of, 28, 128, 130-137
    in Vietnam, 150
  creativity and, 76-77
  crime and, 95-111, 128-144
  etymological origins, 14
  in food, 72-73
  heroin and, 79-94
  history of, 3-14
  medical aspect, 4, 79-94
  methods of use, 62-78
  Mexico as a producer of, 128-136
  pharmacology of, 43-61
  physical addiction, 56-57, 58, 87-88
  physical effects, 43-61
  the plant, 34-42
    appearance of, 35
    classification of, 34-35
    two forms of, 35
  preparation of, 38
  psychic effects, 43-61
  religious use, 4, 13-14
  rolling a cigarette, 70, 71
  in the U.S., ix, xi-xii, xiii, 13, 14, 15-33, 36-37, 42, 53, 57-61, 63-64, 70, 71, 73
    the authorities and, 112-127

Boston University report, 43, 54-57, 60
criminal aspects, 95-111, 128-144
five main groups purchasing, 129
heroin and, 79-94
La Guardia Report, 27-28, 36, 41, 42-54, 58-60, 70, 73-75, 83-87, 89, 97, 99, 104, 107, 134, 137-138
legalization aspect, xi, 26, 31-33, 42, 60, 77-78, 93-94, 110, 111, 122, 125-127
medical aspects, 79-94
military aspects, 145-152
number of users, 31, 63
various names for, 3
world-wide usage, 5
Marijuana: America's New Drug Problem (Walton), 53, 57, 80-82, 131
"Marijuana Bugaboo, The" (Phelan), 147
"Marijuana: Factor in Personality Evaluation and Army Maladjustment" (Friedman and Rockmore), 84
Marijuana: Myths and Realities (Simmons), 63, 110-111
Marijuana Newsletter, 36
"Marijuana: A Psychiatric Study" (Bromberg), 87-88, 98-99
Marijuana Tax Act of 1937, 16, 26, 27, 37, 41, 43, 118, 119
"Marijuana Use in Vietnam: A Preliminary Report," 148
Marriage, 226-228
Masters, Dr. R. E. L., xiii-xiv, 190-193, 200, 201, 230
Mayas, 13-14
Medico-Legal Journal, 254
Memory test, 49
Mencken, H. L., 77
Mendoza, Niño, 131
Mental health, LSD and, 214-224
Mescaline, 11, 57, 58, 110, 122, 175
Methamphetamine hydrochloride, 239, 240
Methedrine, xiv, 54, 194, 239-255, 257
cost, 258, 261-262
Mexican-Americans, 14, 22-23, 129, 135
Mexico, 13, 14, 22-23, 28, 37, 38, 42, 53, 70, 71, 128, 162, 165-167, 181
as a producer of marijuana, 128-136
Michaux, 57
Middle East, 3, 5, 13, 37, 38, 44, 73, 112
Mikuriva, Dr. Tod M., 82-83
Miles ataximeter, 48
Military Surgeon, 147
Milltown, 234
Moore, Harley, Jr., 148
Morning-glory seeds, 183
Morphine, 26, 42, 83, 90, 249
Moslems, 5-6
Mota, 22-23
Motion pictures, 30, 63
Mount, Ferdinand, 77-78
Mouse Studios, 71
Murphy, Dr. H. B., 100, 109
Music, 30, 31, 63-64
Myself and I (Newland), 228-229

Napoleon I, 7, 112
"Narcotic Problem, The: A Brief Study—1965," 97
Narcotics: Nature's Dangerous Gifts (Taylor), 3-4
National Association of Police Officers, 126
National Coordinating Council on Drug Abuse Education and Information, 185
National Institute of Mental Health, 82, 192
National Review, 77, 125-126
Native American Church, 175, 176
Negroes, 23, 28, 29, 30, 32, 74-75, 84, 92-93, 109, 123, 129, 135, 210
Neo-American Church, 175
New Republic, The (magazine), 31, 127
New Statesman, The, 31
New York Academy of Medicine, 27-28, 44
New York Civil Liberties Union, 125
New York Post, 184
New York State Council on Drug Addiction, 93
New York Times, The, 56, 89, 91-92, 93, 94
Newland, Constance, 228-229
Newspapers, 24, 26, 30, 31-32, 63, 85, 101, 124, 132-133, 164, 165
Newsweek (magazine), 32-33, 184
Nureyev, Rudolf, 31
Nutmeg, 235

On the Trial of Marihuana (booklet), 89
Opium, 26, 72, 83, 112-113, 117, 149
Opium Advisory Association, 25
Opium pipes, 72
Osmond, Dr. Humphrey, 218, 222, 223
Oswald, Dr. I., 245
Oteri, Joseph S., 126-127

Palma, Rafael, 130
Panama Canal Zone, 145-147
Panama Canal Zone's Governor's Committee, 146
Paregoric, 112
Pep pills, 239
Periwinkle leaves, 236
Peyote, 11, 42, 57, 59, 110, 122, 175
Pharmacology (Drill), 183
Phelan, James M., 147
Phenyl-2-propanone, 260-261
Pick-up smoking, 74
Pipes, 72
  water, 72
Poland, 40
Popular press, the, 24, 26, 30-33, 63, 85, 101, 122, 124, 132-133, 164, 165, 176
Portugal, 14
Postell, Wilfred, 148
Potheads, 66-70, 71-72, 74
Powelson, Dr. David H., 77
Preminger, Otto, 30-31
President's Commission on Crime, 31
President's Commission on Law Enforcement, 80
Pressy X-O test, 50
Prohibition, 113-114
Psilocin, 175
Psilocybin, 122, 163, 165, 175
Psychedelic Review, 229-230
Puerto Ricans, 84-85, 92-93, 129, 135, 136
Pushers, 88-89, 101, 135-137
  college students, 138-141
Pyle's digit-symbol test, 49

Quinlan, Lawrence, 168

Radio, 63
Rawlin, John W., 252
Report of the Indian Hemp Drug Commission, 44
Rinkel, Dr. Max, 158-159, 216
Ritalin, 194
Roach holders, 72
Roaches, 71-72
Robinson, Dr. Victor, 82
Rockefeller, Nelson, 125
Rockmore, 84
Rolling Stones, 31
Rorschach test, 50
Rosenthal, Dr. M., 121
Ross, Dr. J., 223
Rothlin, Dr. Ernst, 160
Russia, 16

Sadomasochism, 230
Sandoz Chemical Works, 155, 156, 160
Sandox Pharmaceuticals, 182, 237
Sargent, Dr. William, 241
Saturday Evening Post (magazine), 89, 163
Scandinavia, 158
Schizophrenia, 217-218, 243-244, 250-251
Science (magazine), 54-56, 186
Scotch Broom plant, 236
Set and setting, 187-190
Sex, 114, 122
  amphetamines and, 255
  LSD and, 200, 225-230
  marijuana and, 102-104
Shen Neng, 3, 4
"Should We Legalize Pot?" (magazine article), 31
Siberia, 4
Sidle, Winant, 148
Sigma Chemical Company, 182
Silvergate, Harvey A., 126-127
Simmons, J. L., 63
Sleeping pills, 233, 234, 256
Smith, Dr. David, 107, 247
Sniffing, 235
South African Medical Journal, 98
Spain, 6-7, 14, 71, 240
Spanish Civil War, 240
Spectator, The, 31
Speed, 239, 256-262
  See also Amphetamines
Stanley, Owsley, 184-185
Stashing, 69-70
Stein, Gertrude, 72-73
Steinbeck, John, IV, 148
Stewart, William, 185
Stoll, Dr. Arthur, 155, 158
STP, 179, 185, 237, 260

Stuart, Dr. William M., 105
Switzerland, 155-158
Synhexyl, 41

Taiwan, 258
Talbott, Strobe, 32
Task Force on Narcotics and Drug Abuse, 121-122
Taylor, Norman, 3-4
Tea, marijuana, 73
Tea pads, 74-75, 137
Television, 30, 63
Tetrahydrocannabinol (THC), 40
Thackore, V. R., 245
Thailand, 117, 149
Thematic-apperception test, 50
Therapeutic Gazette, 102
Tibetan Book of the Dead, x
Time (magazine), 31, 90-91
Tobacco, 79, 104-105, 107, 108, 112
Toklas, Alice B., 73
Tonight Show (TV), 30
Tours, Dr. Moreau de, 7
Toward a Rational View of Marijuana (McGlothlin), 110-111
"Traffic in Opium and Other Dangerous Drugs" (report), 115
Tranquilizers, 194-195, 233, 234, 237, 256
Transvestism, 230
Treasury Department, 45, 115
Treatment of Drug Addiction: Experience in India (Chopra and Chopra), 85
Trethowan, W. H., 248-249, 254-255
Tryptamines, 237
"Two Cases of Cannabis Indica Intoxication," 102

Unger, Dr. Sanford, 223-224
United Nations, 5, 117
United Nations Commission on Narcotic Drugs, 259
United Nations Single Convention on Narcotic Drugs, 117, 119
United Nations Single Narcotics and Drug Act, 130
United States, 40
  amphetamines, 233-238, 251-254, 256-262
  the current scene in, ix-xiv
  LSD, 158-160, 178-186
    antilegislation, 171-177
    the Leary-Alpert complex, 161-170
    number of users, 180
  marijuana in, ix, xi-xii, xiii, 13, 14, 15-33, 36-37, 42, 53, 57-61, 63-64, 70, 71, 73
    the authorities and, 112-127
    Boston University report, 43, 54-57, 60
    criminal aspects, 95-111, 128-144
    five main groups purchasing, 129
    heroin and, 79-94
    La Guardia Report, 27-28, 36, 41, 42-54, 58-60, 70, 73-75, 83-87, 89, 97, 99, 104, 107, 134, 137-138
    legalization aspect, xi, 26, 31-33, 42, 60, 77-78, 93-94, 110-111, 122, 125-127
    medical aspects, 79-94
    military aspects, 145-152
    number of users, 31, 63
  opium, 112-113
United States Army Medical Corps, 146
United States Pharmacopoeia, 43
Use of Cannabis Drugs in India, The (Chopra and Chopra), 85

Vanishing Adolescent, The (Friedenberg), 108
Varieties of Psychedelic Experience, The (Masters and Houston), xiii-xiv
Viet Cong, 149, 150
Vietnam, 147-152, 256
Vietnam Medical Bulletin, 148
Vinblastine, 236
Vincristin, 236
Volstead Act, 113, 167-170

Wall Street Journal, 90
Walton, Dr. R. P., 53, 57, 80-82, 103, 131
Washington, George, 16
Weber, Father Carlo, 108
Wechsler free-association test, 50
Wechsler vocational-interest test, 50
Weil, Andrew T., 54-57
West, Dr. Louis, 159
West Indies, 39, 82

"What Is So Bad About Marijuana," 118
Whipple steadiness tester, 48
White, James R., 125
White Cross, 88-89
White House Conference on Narcotics and Drug Abuse, 121
"Wild Grass Chase, The" (Mount), 77
Wingmothe, Donna, 173-174
Wood, H. C., 103
World Health Organization (WHO), 106, 117, 259, 260
World War II, 16-17, 147, 240, 256
Wyzanski, Judge Charles, 90

Yale Daily News, 32
Yale Review, 80
Yolles, Dr. Stanley, 238
Young Americans for Reagan, 125
Yugoslavia, 40

Zinberg, Dr. Norman E., 54-55